Praise for
THE SECRET LIFE OF FAT

"You can outsmart your body fat, but first you must understand it! With the right lifestyle, eating, and exercise approach you can lose weight and keep it off. Learn how in this engaging and informative masterpiece."
　　　　　—Michael Dansinger, MD, MS, founding director of the
　　　　　Diabetes Reversal Program at Tufts Medical Center

"For years we presumed that body fat is just a depot for energy, but current science is proving that it is actually the largest endocrine gland in our body. This enigmatic organ conveys many paradoxes and surprises; depending on its location, color, and genetic makeup, it might be either dangerous or protective."
　　　　　—Osama Hamdy, medical director of the Obesity
　　　　　Clinical Program at Joslin Diabetes Center,
　　　　　and author of *The Diabetes Breakthrough*

"This book by Dr. Sylvia Tara addresses important concepts related to the pathogenesis, prevention, and treatment of obesity with attention directed at the past, present, and future. A very interesting read for lay people interested in fat and obesity, as well as for many in the scientific community."
　　　　　—Carl Lavie, MD, clinician and scientist in cardiovascular
　　　　　prevention, and author of *The Obesity Paradox*

"A refreshing change to the conflicting advice and opinions about food that we are subjected to every day."
　　　　　—Philippa Matthews, *Chemistry World*

"Powerful . . . [Tara's] research and insight are deeply perspective-shifting."
　　　　　—Melissa Wuske, *Foreword*

"Like comfort food for anyone carrying around a lifetime of guilt for eating an extra cookie."
—Hadassah

"Finally, a book that sheds some light on understanding body fat—specifically, its role, why it is so difficult to fight, and how it works differently for different people. . . . This genuinely enlightening book will be a revelation to those engulfed in self-blame and shame about their weight."
—Publishers Weekly

THE SECRET LIFE OF
FAT

*The Science Behind the Body's Least Understood Organ
and What It Means for You*

THE
SECRET LIFE OF
FAT

Sylvia Tara, PhD

W. W. NORTON & COMPANY
Independent Publishers Since 1923
New York · London

For information about permission to reproduce selections from this book,
write to Permissions, W. W. Norton & Company, Inc.,
500 Fifth Avenue, New York, NY 10110

For information about special discounts for bulk purchases, please contact
W. W. Norton Special Sales at specialsales@wwnorton.com or 800-233-4830

Manufacturing by Quad Graphics, Fairfield
Book design by Charlotte Staub
Production manager: Louise Mattarelliano

Library of Congress Cataloging-in-Publication Data

Names: Tara, Sylvia.
Title: The secret life of fat : the science behind the body's least understood
organ and what it means for you / Sylvia Tara, PhD.
Description: First edition. | New York : W.W. Norton & Company, [2017] |
Includes bibliographical references and index.
Identifiers: LCCN 2016027841 | ISBN 9780393244830 (hardcover)
Subjects: LCSH: Fat. | Fat—Health aspects.
Classification: LCC QP752.F3 T37 2017 | DDC 613.2—dc23 LC record
available at https://lccn.loc.gov/2016027841

ISBN 978-0-393-35497-3 pbk.

W. W. Norton & Company, Inc.
500 Fifth Avenue, New York, N.Y. 10110
www.wwnorton.com

W. W. Norton & Company Ltd.
15 Carlisle Street, London W1D 3BS

1 2 3 4 5 6 7 8 9 0

The Secret Life of Fat *is a work of nonfiction. With the exception of those whose stories have been reported elsewhere, or who have agreed to be identified here, the individuals whose struggles appear in these pages are referred to by aliases, and some of their identifying characteristics have been changed. Where my own story is concerned, I ask the reader to bear in mind that my approach is not for everyone. No book can replace the expertise of a trained professional who has examined you and is familiar with your medical history. Please be certain to consult with your physician before making changes to your current food or exercise regimen, particularly if you are pregnant, suffer from any medical condition, or have any symptoms that may require treatment.*

Dedicated to my parents

CONTENTS

Prologue—Skinny Jeans ix
Introduction—Our Changing Views of Fat 1

I. All About Fat

1. The Foundation: Fat Does More Than You Think 11
2. Fat Can Talk 26
3. Your Life Depends on Fat 46
4. When Good Fat Goes Bad 63
5. How Fat Fights to Stay on You 78

II. It Is Not Only Food That Makes Us Fat

6. Bacteria and Viruses—Microscopic in Size, Giant in Effect 97
7. I Blame My Parents—Genes in Obesity 121
8. I Am Woman, I Have Fat 132
9. Fat Can Listen 146

III. So What Is the Solution?

10. Fat Control I: How You Can Do It 165
11. Mind over Fat 179
12. Fat Control II: How I Do It 191
13. The Future of Fat 202

Acknowledgments 209
Bibliography and References 211
Index 225

Prologue

Skinny Jeans

It was a breezy Friday evening in the fall in San Diego. I was a biochemistry PhD student out to dinner with friends after a full week of research, classes, and teaching. I'd had a strong interest in biology since grade school, particularly in how the body malfunctions and the inventive ways we treat it. The idea that tiny molecules affected our health, thoughts, and quality of life was fascinating to me.

Though I was excited to be learning so much about the inner workings of the body, another interest tugged at me constantly— my weight. Aside from advancing my career, I measured success in how well I did at staying thin. Keeping my fat in check had never been easy for me, and I watched my weight closely. On this day, like every other, I had counted my calories since morning. I ate a painstakingly balanced combination of grains, proteins, and vegetables. I abstained from anything fun—no sugar, carb-heavy snacks, or alcohol. I had run for forty minutes, and lifted weights. After months of this diligent work, I knew I was on my way towards fitness victory.

As I sat down to dinner with my friends, I held steadfast—I ordered a small salad and water. Like so many days before, I was bracing to go to bed hungry. Going to bed hungry was my secret to keeping my five-foot-three-inch frame under 110 pounds and capable of fitting into skinny jeans. If I could just maintain this weight, my life would remain in my control, I'd look like every other college student, I'd be asked out on dates, and I'd feel confident about my future.

But instead of feeling proud of my dieting achievement that night, something happened that would forever change the way I viewed my body. Something profound, that confirmed I was not "normal."

What happened? My friend ordered a beer and burrito and devoured it all. Yes, that seemingly trivial event changed everything.

Lindsey was four foot eleven inches and probably about 95 pounds. She never went to the gym. She drank sugary lattes and indiscriminately ate fast food. She worked in the lab all day like me, and hunched over a computer in the evening. Yet somehow this petite woman was able to pack in a large steak burrito, with beans, rice, sour cream, guacamole, cheddar cheese all wrapped in a flour tortilla, and then down a beer as if all this were nothing unusual. She had no guilt afterward, no appearance of worry, she made no comments about feeling sick after eating it or how she would need to run on the treadmill the next morning. Nothing. It was all just a normal everyday occurrence to eat an 800-calorie dinner at eight o'clock in the evening. And her jeans were smaller than mine!

How could this be? I lived with ongoing hunger, pain, and discipline to stay thin. If I ever took one step out of line, I had to pay a price on the scale. Yet, here was this effortlessly tiny woman who ate three times what I would ever dare to consume in one sitting. I felt as though nature was cackling in my face—"Look how unfair I can be and how little you can do about it."

This was one of the moments in my life that made me realize that we are *not* all created equal, at least not when it comes to fat. Just as some people are taller, or produce more sweat, or grow more hair, there are some who simply produce more fat than others. And one of those people happened to be me. Although the burrito incident forced me to face this realization, I had actually suspected something was amiss long before.

As a child, I always had some extra abdominal fat. I didn't realize it was extra until I was nine, when at a summer pool party my friends showed up in their bikinis. I noticed they all had flat bellies and clearly visible ribs in contrast to my softer midsection. I didn't give it too much thought at the time. But as puberty approached, I started gaining more weight. In addition to developing curves and oily skin, I started packing on fat.

At age twelve, I conscientiously went on my first diet, to lose ten pounds. While my friends were eating ice cream all summer, I studied nutrition and employed military-like discipline on my 1,000-calorie daily limit. I weighed myself diligently and started losing a pound a week. I was feeling good, until one week late in August.

With summer ending I was almost at my target weight, so I thought I'd loosen up a bit. I accepted half a piece of licorice from my friend, who went on to consume the rest of the pack. When I got on the scale for my weekly weigh-in, not only did I not lose a pound, I had actually gained two. It was demoralizing to say the least. How could half a piece of candy do so much damage? How was it that my friends ate without reservation, and I was forced to scrutinize every calorie if I wanted to look like them? I stayed careful about food, but didn't lose more than eight pounds that summer.

Throughout high school my weight moved in fits and starts. I'd reach my ideal weight and then I'd suddenly be ten pounds over. It was never easy. As I became close to other girls, they confided that they experienced similar problems with fat. Their eyes would well with tears as they talked about their weight struggles. There was so much pressure to be thin. There were girls who turned bulimic, and those who started doing drugs as a way to keep their weight down. Maintaining "thin" in the teenage years was not a light undertaking for everyone.

Magazines tell us that if we follow their simple suggestions to "eat right" and exercise, we will look like the models they display. How many headlines tantalize us with "Lose Belly Fat in 5 Days," "Eat Whole Grains And Burn Fat," "Simple Exercise Regimen For Thinner Thighs"? All, of course, accompanied by images of young, fit models, although we have no idea how they really got that way. The messages insinuate that if we are not thin it is our own fault; the rules are easy to follow. And it isn't just magazines, but the massive diet industry that feeds us the hope of being skinny, and blames us if we are not.

Today we spend an enormous amount of time and money on the promise of being thin. People are constantly reminded that fat is a problem, they have it, and they need to get rid of it. Yet, for all of our efforts, the obesity rate keeps growing. The truth is that managing fat is by far more complicated than magazines lead you to believe.

Some brave individuals have spoken out about the intense battle they fight to look "normal." Actress Lisa Rinna told *People* magazine she starves herself on the days she needs to wear a formfitting gown for awards. She also takes appetite suppressants in order to eat just enough "to keep going." Cindy Crawford has spoken about how easily she gained weight compared to other models. In her photos she sometimes appeared fleshier than the skinny models posing alongside of her. She followed a low-carb diet plan, and had the financial means to hire experts to help her stay thin. Valerie Bertinelli has written about actresses going on strict diets before auditions, only to go back to eating and packing on flesh once the filming is over. Apparently, even those we envy for their thinness go through much more than we know to get that way.

For me, being thin was always more work than it was for others. I put up a good fight through graduate school and my early career and succeeded at wearing my skinny jeans into my thirties. But once kids came along, I started gaining weight. During my first pregnancy, I had the typical twenty-pound gain. With my second child came another ten pounds. I noticed the same weight gain on a number of my career-minded friends who also had children. It seemed that the stress of a full-time job, young children waking up through the night, and the new responsibility for managing it all pushed weight control onto the back burner. All I could think about was trying to juggle everything and make it through the day.

As my kids got older, and I got my new life under control, I reengaged in the battle to fight fat and hired a personal trainer named David. His technique borrowed from the new philosophy of weight loss in which you need to eat enough calories and exercise in order to shed pounds. The thinking is that if you eat insufficiently, the body goes into starvation mode and hoards every calorie, making weight loss much harder (this same philosophy appears on the show

The Biggest Loser.) David required that I keep a log of everything I ate, and that I made sure to have a balance of carbohydrates, vegetables, and protein paired with a two-hours-a-day exercise regime. He reviewed my food log after the first week and was aghast at how few calories I was taking in—around 1,200. He swore that given my height and muscle mass, I needed to add a few hundred more calories per day in order to lose weight.

I obliged, and immediately started gaining fat. After three weeks, David admitted that his theory of increasing calories was not working for me, and I went back to my 1,200 calories per day. I always recognized that my body turned food into fat more readily than other people's did, but for some this is hard to believe. I lost weight with David, but in the end two hours per day of exercise wasn't feasible, so I reverted to a few hours of exercise a week, and lived with some extra fat. All the while my husband and kids ate abundantly and had no trouble staying thin.

As time went on I started to get more annoyed with my fat, particularly as I observed that some women who also had children and a career and exercised only occasionally appeared to have less fat than I did. I began noticing everything about fat. Mine looked different; it was softer and more fluid. On business trips with colleagues, eating late at night would cause my flesh to expand more than anyone else's. I could gain almost five pounds in a week just by eating dinners. The difference in fat among people was fascinating to me. Fat seemed to have a mind of its own.

The final provocation came one day after an exercise class. I joined aerobics with a friend, Laura, who was in her early forties, had three kids and a job, and was model thin. I was impressed with her ability to stay so slender and wondered how she did it. We both pounded out a good sweat in our class and still prudently ordered salads for lunch. As we sat and chatted, I ate half of mine and saved the remainder for dinner, as I often did. Dividing one lunch into two meals was my new secret for preventing my weight from rising even higher. But Laura kept eating. She ate every bit of the large chicken salad she ordered, and then had nuts and a sugary coffee afterward.

I asked Laura what she usually had for dinner. She said she ate what her kids were having—tacos, chicken, steak, whatever. Hold on, I thought. *Whatever?* We are the same age, in the same exercise class, have the same career demands, and have multiple children. Yet she eats almost double what I do and is half my size?

I'd had it. This was the burrito story all over again. This was the licorice story all over again. This was the final observation that I couldn't ignore. I was fed up with watching everyone around me eat more, choose foods indiscriminately, exercise sporadically, and yet have less fat than I did. There must be something more to weight gain besides "eating right" and exercising. There must be . . . something else, something besides the typical everyday assumptions we all make about the nature of fat.

This brought me full circle back to graduate school. When I was a biochemistry PhD candidate, the natural next step was to start a career in research, but I felt conflicted. An advisor gave me this advice: if you don't have a burning question for which you need to find the answer, don't go into research. It was sound guidance as a postdoctoral fellowship entails long hours, low pay, and years of inherent uncertainty. I didn't have a burning question at the time, so I entered the business side of science instead. But now, more than a decade later, I had that burning question: why was it easier for some people to stay thin than others? How did fat work? Furthermore, why did food affect people in different ways? Why was fat harder to control with age? I needed to understand fat once and for all.

I was a scientist by training, and if anyone was capable of getting to the bottom of this, I was. If observation is the first step of the scientific method, I'd had more than enough. From this day forward, I promised myself, I would devote every available moment to understanding fat. The chapters that follow are what I found out about the secret life of fat.

THE SECRET LIFE OF
FAT

Introduction

Our Changing Views
of Fat

After skillfully guiding his party to landmark election wins in 1994, Newt Gingrich was deemed one of the most powerful people in the United States. He had overcome what seemed like an insurmountable hurdle—uniting warring factions of the Republican Party and creating the comprehensive Contract with America. His strategy redefined the conservative agenda and helped his party win back the House of Representatives for the first time since 1954.

In an interview with Barbara Walters for her annual prime-time special, *The 10 Most Fascinating People of 1995*, the probing host asked her usual assortment of personal questions. Finally, she came to her specialty, the one guaranteed to make her subject squirm: "What do you like least about yourself?"

A suspenseful pause followed. Was Gingrich going to say his failed marriage, his contentious involvement with scandals, the questionable political decisions he had made in his past? He did not.

"I'm most embarrassed about my weight," he said.

"Aww," Walters said, trying to ease the awkwardness.

He went on, "I know it's entirely a function of my personality that I swim, I eat the right things, and then I either have a chance to drink some Guinness or to eat some ice cream, and I cave."

It was an unforgettable TV moment. Even for the man standing at the pinnacle of power, what hurt him the most on the inside? His fat.

Poor fat! So reviled, so shameful, so unloved. It betrays our glut-tony, our lack of self-control, our low self-esteem, our abject unwor-thiness. We want only to annihilate it, or at least keep it to a barely visible minimum. We spend billions trying to banish it by investing in diet foods, books, exercise clubs, drugs, counselors, and medical treatments. In fact, we spend more on the war on fat than the war on terror—$44.7 billion was budgeted for U.S. Homeland Security in 2014, but about $60 billion was spent fighting fat. And this does not include the $1 billion spent each year on ads promoting products that promise all of us a better life if only we could only rid ourselves of our fat. We are indeed a nation at war with a body part.

But fat remains unvanquished. In fact you could say fat is bigger than ever: more than 78 million Americans are considered obese and millions more, overweight; almost half of Germans are overweight, and people in the United Kingdom, Hungary, and Australia are not too far behind.

Though fat is reviled around the globe, the truth is it is simply an organ in our body. That's right—an *organ*. This comes as a surprise to many who think fat is merely blubber. But new research is show-ing us that fat is part of the endocrine system, and scientists have been referring to it as an organ for years. It turns out that fat may be just as important as our colon, lungs, and heart.

Fat accommodates our everyday energy needs for things such as walking, talking, running, and even sleeping. Fat is there to make sure every bodily function continues when we skip lunch to meet a deadline, fast for religious purposes, or simply don't feel like cooking dinner. It is also there for us when we eat even one more ounce of food than we actually need. If you ever gave in to a dessert that was too tantalizing to pass up, be thankful fat was ready and waiting to absorb it. Fat acts like the body's central bank, managing excess and providing resources when needed. It is willing to expand itself in times of feast and selflessly cannibalize itself in times of need to keep other organs alive.

Fat not only does the enormous job of managing our energy

stores; research is revealing that it also enables puberty, allows our reproductive organs to function, strengthens bones, enhances our immune system, and even boosts our brain size (think of that next time you call someone a fathead!).

Though it is now the target of a multibillion dollar offensive, fat was not always hated. It was once humankind's admired companion. Our nomadic ancestors welcomed it as a cushion against bouts of starvation. Even as civilizations evolved through the centuries, fat held a special place. Buddha's fat has remained his signature—it's a major part of his brand, you could say. In China during the Tang Dynasty (AD 618–907), tombstone sculptures depicted plump women in the belief they would help the dead find prosperity in the afterlife. More recently, Botticelli, Rubens, and Titian all depicted fat as necessary to the beautiful human form. The standards for thinness that are celebrated in *Vogue* today are nowhere to be found in the past, unless it was to portray suffering.

Even in America, there was a time when fat was respected. After the Civil War, poverty increased dramatically, but a small segment of society managed to thrive. As with everything else that is precious and scarce in the world, like gold or gems, when fat was hard to obtain, its value soared. Fat was a sign of prosperity, health, and beauty. Everyone wanted it.

It may be hard to believe, but the evidence of the time supports our love of fat. A prestigious group called the Fat Man's Club was founded in Connecticut in 1866, espousing the saying, "A fat bank account tends to make a fat man." Men were required to be stout enough to join. Women also prided themselves on fleshiness, consulting the *Ladies Home Journal* on how to gain weight or the 1878 book *How To Be Plump*. Instead of trying to fit into size 0, celebrities were praised for poundage. Singer Lillian Russell weighed over two hundred pounds and was admired for her flesh as much as her voice. Women even padded themselves to look like her. And Diamond Jim Brady, the Donald Trump of his day, was loved not only for his wealth but also for his weight (three hundred pounds).

Even physicians supported fat. They cautioned against obesity, but suggested gaining some pounds as a way to treat nervousness and even contagious disease. Parents also encouraged their kids to eat amply.

These were good times for fat. It was appreciated for its positive qualities—to supply energy and symbolize well-being. But sadly for the organ, its heyday didn't last. As America's economy improved, food became more accessible—and so did fat. As with any resource, when there is plenty of it, it is no longer precious. Fat's value sank.

Now business leaders stressed the need for efficient and thin bodies for the labor force. Military leaders linked leanness to love of country; said one, "Any healthy, normal individual who is now getting fat is unpatriotic." And religious leaders reinforced fat as a reflection of excess and gluttony. Physicians, treating a more fat-conscious clientele, also started doling out advice on how to lose weight. Celebrities, including Lillian Russell, got caught in the twist and were forced to reduce their size. And the Fat Man's Club, a sign of affluence in previous years, closed its doors in 1903.

The attention to fat started out as well-intended caution against the country's growing girth, but it soon turned to disdain. Slurs like "fat slob" and "fatty" found their way into everyday conversation. Cartoons poking fun at the obese appeared in print. Even the president of the United States, 305-pound Howard Taft, couldn't escape ridicule. One headline read, "Taft Causes Hotel Deluge: Tidal Wave from his Bathtub Floods Bankers in Dining Room." The "Taft Tub" tale lived on for years afterward.

A landmark in weight obsession was the introduction of the calorie to measure nutrition. The calorie was defined in the 1800s as the amount of energy needed to raise the temperature of one kilogram of water by one degree Celsius. Then at the end of the century, Wilbur Atwater performed detailed studies on how our bodies use food for energy by putting test subjects in a closed chamber and evaluating the amount of carbon dioxide they produced as well as the level of oxygen they consumed after eating various foods. He translated his findings into energy units, and the calorie became the standard measurement of food value. In 1918, physician Lulu Hunt Peters called counting calories an active form of patriotism and published *Diet and Health: With*

Key to the Calories, selling two million copies—likely the first diet best seller. The business of dieting was afoot.

As time went on, weight-loss advice became more exploitive, taking advantage of the nation's growing fears about fat. Opportunists introduced several gimmicks, hoping to make a quick profit. Rubber suits were sold that would supposedly help people sweat away weight. The Gardner Reducing Machine claimed that applying pressure to skin would massage away fat. "Fatoff" and "La Mar Reducing Soap" were introduced in the 1930s, claiming to dissolve fat under the skin. A few individuals got rich, but fat remained.

Questionable diets were contrived, too. Some companies saw the dieting craze as a means to increase revenue. In the 1920s Lucky Strike Cigarettes advertised, "Reach for a Lucky instead of a sweet." The campaign worked and sales of the cigarettes grew by 200 percent. The Grapefruit Diet was introduced and required eating a grapefruit with every meal in the belief that the fruit contains a powerful fat-burning enzyme. The Drinking Man's Diet claimed that since vodka, gin, and whiskey had only traces of carbohydrate, they were okay to drink freely. Typical meals included steak with fattening sauces, and a glass of liquor to wash it down. The book sold 2.4 million copies in two years, and was translated into thirteen languages.

Entrepreneurs looked for any way to sell fat loss. In 1933, physicians at Stanford University noticed that dinitrophenol (DNP), an ingredient in explosives, increased metabolism by causing an increase in body heat. Soon after, DNP was available in the market for losing fat and had predictably dangerous side effects, including death and blindness. Deaths from DNP are still being reported (as recently as 2015) as desperate dieters continue to seek fast weight loss. Dieters even swallowed live tapeworm eggs believing that the parasites, once hatched, would consume food eaten by the host and prevent fat. Once the desired weight was achieved, the dieter would swallow poison to kill the tapeworms. It sounds like a horror movie—incubating three-yard-long worms in your intestines and then imbibing poison cocktails. But to some, it was better than carrying a few extra pounds.

As the nation became more corporate, so did dieting. Starting in the 1960s, large multinationals took over from the peddlers of home-spun diet aids. Weight Watchers, Nutrisystem, and Jenny Craig took weight control mainstream. With organized business behind it, the dieting industry exploded.

Today, fighting fat has even become a spectator sport. *The Biggest Loser* reality show, considered a gamble when it first aired, is now one of the most successful shows on television. Its founder, JD Roth, says that in the beginning securing contestants was more difficult than for other game shows because obese people were embarrassed to take part. Roth recalls, "I remember trying to get staff to work on the show. I had an entire lunchroom room full of editors and story people. I would say more than half of them said that they didn't want to be on the show." He says, "There was so much embarrass-ment around the whole idea of overweight people in reality shows."

Seventeen seasons later, *The Biggest Loser* attracts an average of 6 million viewers and has spawned about a dozen more shows to exploit the same combination of dread and fascination we have with body fat. We've had *Fat Actress* (Kirstie Alley), *Heavy* (extreme obe-sity), *One Big Happy Family*, *Love Handles* (fat couples), *Shedding for the Wedding*, *Dance Your A** Off*, *DietTribe*, *I Used to Be Fat*, with millions tuning in. JD Roth even launched another show, *Extreme Makeover: Weight Loss Edition*, featuring people too obese for *The Biggest Loser*.

How could the echo chamber urging fat's obliteration not affect how we think of ourselves—and one another—if we have the mis-fortune to put on a pound or three? Though caution against obesity is well placed, treating fat like a vicious enemy is not. We spend billions in the war against fat—chemical weapons, surgical devices, behavior restructuring, exercise contraptions, and rationed food programs—but despite our best efforts, fat returns.

Clearly, we do not understand the enemy we're fighting. Metabo-lism is far more complicated than the simple arithmetic of a calorie in, a calorie out. We are not pure calorie-burning machines. We are an intricate system of biology, hormones, genetics, and bacteria pro-cessing nutrients individually. Obviously, we'll need a much deeper understanding of fat if we are to control it.

And maybe as we start to understand our "enemy" we'll realize that it is not all bad. New research is showing us that fat secretes essential hormones, enables many bodily functions, keeps us safe from disease, and may even help us live longer. Fat appears to be so important that our stem cells are capable of creating it independent of our food intake—a function that has been observed for critical tissues such as muscle, bone, and brain.

Perhaps nature does have reasons to keep fat on us, despite all our attempts to remove it, which may bring us to another twist in the saga of fat. With all its newly discovered talents, fat could become beloved once again. And if that is the case, then maybe Newt Gingrich had less to be embarrassed about than he thought.

Certainly, he's not alone in his shame. Nearly two decades after Gingrich's confession, Barbara Walters's unerring instinct for emotional frailty had the same effect on another subject. In 2014, she interviewed Oprah Winfrey. After steering her guest through the highs and lows of her career and personal life, Walters arrived at the pivotal moment. She asked Winfrey to complete this sentence: "Before I leave this earth I will not be satisfied until I. . . ."

Winfrey started, "Until . . . ," then paused, ". . . I make peace with the whole weight thing."

Walters was incredulous. She leaned forward and yelled, "What?! That's still on your mind? . . . I was expecting something deeply profound."

"No, that's it," Winfrey said. "I've got to make peace with it."

Maybe Oprah's not the only one.

I

ALL ABOUT
FAT

Chapter 1

The Foundation: Fat Does More Than You Think

So what is fat exactly? We all agree that fat, in its simplest form, is a reserve of energy, perhaps a relic from our nomadic ancestors who needed it to protect against frequent famine. But now that there are supermarkets and fast-food chains on every corner, fat seems to be a biological anachronism. Even the dictionary definition of fat—"a natural oily or greasy substance occurring in animal bodies, especially when deposited as a layer under the skin or around certain organs"—reinforces the idea that it is not particularly important to us.

Not reflected in the common understanding, however, is the vast importance fat has in our lives. From managing our energy stores, to enabling transmission of brain signals, to facilitating labor in pregnacy, fat has shown itself to be a critical and versatile body part. Although fat was once thought of as inert blubber, researchers now categorize it as an organ. If you doubt the importance of fat, imagine what would happen if you didn't have any. To get an idea of what life would be like, look no further than the story of Christina Vena.

The Girl with No Fat

Christina was a healthy, vibrant twelve-year-old living in Vineland, New Jersey, in the 1990s. Her days were filled with school, sports, friends, and a newly developing interest in boys. But just as Christina entered puberty, something strange happened. Her body spontaneously began losing fat. Many twelve-year-old girls would rejoice at being a bit skinnier, but Christina's case was worrisome. She lost the fat in her cheeks, hands, and feet. Her looks changed rapidly as her face became sunken and her hands shriveled. Soon, Christina started to lose fat on the rest of her body as well, and her clothes hung off her shrinking frame.

Oddly, at the same time she developed an enormous appetite. She remembers, "I was very hungry. I was hungry to the point where I wouldn't know I was full until I got sick. I ate all of the time, I couldn't stop." Despite all her eating, Christina just kept getting thinner.

Her parents believed she was going through the normal growth spurt of an early teenager. Nothing to worry about, they thought, so they let her eat as much as she wanted. Some of her friends even envied how much Christina could eat and yet stay so thin. But she continued losing fat, and eventually she lost so much that her face became unrecognizable to people who knew her in the past.

It was an unusual pairing—heavy eating coupled with dramatic fat loss. And soon, another strange event took place—bumps started forming on Christina's arms. At first there were just a few soft lumps on her forearms. But eventually, dozens of soft, fluid-filled bumps appeared and wouldn't go away. Her parents grew concerned. They took her to a dermatologist, who ordered blood tests.

The results of the tests were shocking. Christina's total cholesterol was 950 mg/dL, though the normal level for a girl her age is under 170. Her triglycerides, which should have been around 150 mg/dL, measured 16,000. Postmeal blood sugar would normally be 100 mg/dL. Instead, hers was 500. Her blood was literally full of fat, cholesterol, and sugar.

Once Christina's dermatologist reviewed the test results he recognized that this was not a dermatology issue but a metabolic one. He immediately referred Christina to an endocrinologist at the Children's Hospital of Philadelphia.

At first, her endocrinologist thought she had diabetes and started treating her for that. But Christina's health didn't improve. Even as she took her diabetes medicine, her weight continued to drop and her appetite grew. Christina recalls, "I actually would eat anything in the house. It didn't have to be something that tasted great. I would eat anything I could get my hands on, like a can of mushrooms. It was out of control. My parents used to lock the pantry. They put locks on everything, and I would sit there and cry."

The bumps on Christina's arms started spreading. Now they appeared everywhere, from the tips of her toes to her shoulders. Not only were they unsightly, they were inflamed and extremely painful. She says, "If you just touched the bumps, it hurt. And of course, they showed up on all of my pressure points, so I couldn't walk. I had a hard time bathing myself. I had a hard time eating and holding silverware. I had to have special silverware to eat. Just moving in general was starting to be too much."

Her endocrinologist was stumped, until he remembered having heard a lecture given by Dr. Elif Oral at the National Institutes of Health in Bethesda, Maryland. Oral was a specialist in endocrine diseases, diabetes, and metabolic disorders, and was studying patients with symptoms similar to Christina's. The endocrinologist sent Christina to Dr. Oral, who examined her in March 1997.

Dr. Oral recalls, "For us, her fat loss gave away what was happening. By the time we saw her, she had a complete absence of body fat. And because that's what we study, we knew immediately what her problem was." Oral diagnosed Christina with lipodystrophy—a genetic condition that causes body fat to atrophy and ultimately disappear altogether. To confirm the diagnosis, Oral also did a biopsy of Christina's liver, which was greatly enlarged and protruding through her abdomen. She biopsied Christina's kidneys as well, since she had high levels of protein in her urine. All tests confirmed Dr. Oral's diagnosis.

The mystery behind Christina's symptoms—the weight loss and uncontrollable appetite, the high levels of fat in her blood, the soft bumps just under her skin—was finally solved. Without body fat to store the extra nutrients she ate, they circulated endlessly in her bloodstream. There was so much unstored fat that it collected in Christina's liver, greatly enlarging it, and in lumps under her skin, causing the crippling inflammation and pain.

The diagnosis was small comfort, however, because there was no easy treatment for Christina's condition. She routinely underwent plasmapheresis, a process in which her blood was extracted from her body, filtered to remove fats and cholesterol, and reinserted back into her circulation. It was a long, painful, and tiring ordeal she had to undergo up to three times a week.

Worse, there was no cure. Her family was told to start preparing for her death. Christina recalls, "They said there was nothing they could do. I stopped going to school. I just eventually said, you know, if this is going to kill me, I would rather be home . . . We really thought I wasn't going to live, and I was home-schooled for all of high school. It was hard on my parents. My mom was very upset and crying a lot."

The Long Path to Understanding Fat

Christina and her family were learning just how complex the biology of fat can be, and the life-or-death stakes involved when something goes wrong with it. That was shocking enough. Even more surprising, however, is how simplistic our view of fat has been, even in the eyes of medical science.

For centuries, fat was considered simply storage for excess calories, nothing more. Eat a lot and you get chubby; starve and you become thin. But thousands of research studies from around the world are now revealing that fat is not just fat—it is a dynamic and interactive endocrine organ that has life-or-death influence over us. It is so important that nature ensures we have it beginning in the womb. At about fourteen weeks of gestation, the embryo starts to manufacture fat, even before all systems are functioning. As later chapters describe, fat controls our appetite, influences our emotions, supplies energy, and enables the activities of other body parts. No wonder our bodies have multiple means of creating fat, and even more ways of thwarting any attempt to get rid of it.

Scientists have long sought to make sense of fat. The quest to understand it can be traced at least to ancient Greece, where physicians believed that fat was a concoction of congealed blood that occurred more frequently in the "cold" bodies of women. They hypothesized that extra body fluids such as leftover milk from lactation and unused semen were converted into fat, the latter leading to the belief that overweight men were sterile. Hippocrates wrote about fat as "moistness" in the body that could lead to sexual dysfunction if not addressed.

This idea that fat was made from body fluids lived on for many years, though some early scientists and physicians also made the connection between fat, food, and energy. Galen, the Greek physician, touted his ability to use exercise to "reduce a huge fat fellow to a moderate size." King Henry VIII's physician, Dr. Andrew Boorde, blamed sweet wines for the king's fat. Premodern theories about fat focused on food and exercise, a relationship that could be observed with the unaided eye. But it was the development of the microscope in the mid-1600s that deepened our understanding of fat.

In the 1670s, Antonie van Leeuwenhoek successfully produced a lens that could magnify objects over two hundred times their original size. European scientists used van Leeuwenhoek's lenses to examine body fluids, plant elements, pieces of animal organs, and anything else they could fit under the lens. Much to their surprise, they found that plants and animals were composed of small "vesicles." These structures came to be called "cells" and, it was theorized, were the smallest living components of organisms. Scientists learned that cells were self-sustaining bodies that were connected to each other and served as the building blocks of structured organs. When fat was studied under the microscope, it too was found to consist of cells.

What was unique about fat cells, however, was that they had the distinct ability to store fat—lots of it. Fat cells (also called adipocytes) could expand their volume more than one thousand times normal size by pushing other cell contents off to the side.

Cell theory of the seventeenth century was further refined by molecular theory in the nineteenth century. In 1874, Theodore Gobley elucidated the molecular structure of a fat molecule, showing that it is simply a long chain of carbon atoms. Different types of fat molecules were identified and collectively came to be called "lipids."

Piecing these findings together, the scientific community was able to classify the structure of body fat. It is a body part made of fat tissue (also called adipose), composed of fat cells, which store millions of fat molecules that can be used for energy.

| Fat as an organ | Fat, the organ, is made of fat tissue (also known as adipose). | Fat tissue contains individual fat cells (scientifically termed adipocytes). | Fat molecules (or fatty acids) are stored in fat cells. There are many types of fat molecules which are collectively referred to as lipids. |

Over time, it became clear that fat tissue isn't just made of fat. The soft layer that surrounds our bodies was found to be, on average, only three-quarters fat, with the rest composed of collagen fibers that hold it in place; veins and nerves; as well as blood, muscle, and stem and immune cells. When we pinch an inch, we are really not pinching that much fat.

By the twentieth century, scientists were deciphering the process by which our bodies make and use fat. In 1936, Rudolph Schoenheimer and David Rittenberg at Columbia University were able to trace how carbohydrates from food got shuttled to the liver, where a portion was converted into fat molecules. These carbohydrates-turned-fat were then distributed via the bloodstream to fat tissue and deposited there as triglycerides (a triplet form of fat molecules), for long-term storage.

After Schoenheimer and Rittenberg's discovery, researchers believed that the liver made all of the fat in the body. But a decade later, Benyamin Shapiro and Haim Ernst Wertheimer at the Hebrew University of Jerusalem revealed that adipocytes could also make their own fat. Until this time, researchers still believed fat to be mere passive storage with no metabolic capabilities. Shapiro and Wertheimer had discovered that fat possessed the power to produce itself.

A Fat Primer

Eventually, the numerous findings from scientists studying fat—how it's made, where it's stored, how and when our bodies use it—

came together like pieces of a mosaic. A picture emerged showing that the stomach, pancreas, and small intestine break down our food into its components—amino acids, fat, and carbohydrates. These go into the circulatory system, where some get deposited directly into tissues and some go to the liver, where they are broken down and processed further. The liver takes digested food and turns it into substances the body can use for energy, growth, and maintenance. The liver converts a portion of the amino acids we ingest and uses them to create the proteins our bodies need. It takes the remainder of the amino acids, as well as carbohydrates, sugars, and fats, and turns them into three main sources of energy: glucose, glycogen, and fat.

If you want to understand the way our bodies use that energy, think of money. Just as currency is used for every exchange in our economy, energy is needed for every transaction in our bodies. Money exists in different forms: cash, checking accounts, and long-term savings accounts. Sometimes, we need cash to spend right away. Other times we just want it nearby and ready for use. And some we save for that rainy day. In the body, glucose is cash, glycogen is a checking account, and fat is a certificate of deposit.

Glucose, a form of sugar, is like cash because it instantly supplies the body's current energy needs. It is available from food and is also produced by the liver. Hospitals use glucose in drip bags to intravenously feed patients who are unable to eat.

When we have too much cash hanging around, we deposit some into a checking account. In the body, glycogen is that standby reserve—the liver and muscles create glycogen out of glucose, stringing it together in chains and storing it for future use. Once glucose in the bloodstream runs low, our bodies start breaking apart glycogen, one glucose molecule at a time, and burning it as needed.

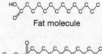
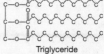

Fat molecule

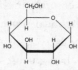

Glucose

Glycogen
(chains of glucose)

Triglyceride

Fat is altogether different. Unlike glycogen, fat is not simply glu-cose stacked away and available for use. Fat molecules (also called fatty acids) are chains of fourteen to twenty carbon atoms that are linked together. These molecules are joined in threes to form tri-glycerides, which are long, lithe, and malleable so they can be packed tightly together in our fat cells. When the body is low on glucose and glycogen, it reaches for fat and converts it into the energy it needs. Fat is the certificate of deposit: not easy to get to, but it can safely hold a lot of energy in reserve.

The scientific term for the process by which our bodies make fat is *lipogenesis*, while the breakdown of fat to release fatty acids into circulation is called *lipolysis*. Lipogenesis occurs most notably after we eat and have excess nutrients to store.

As we digest food, insulin is released from the pancreas and sig-nals cells throughout the body that nourishment is coming, so they should be ready to accept it and either convert it into energy for immediate use or store it. After a meal, our glucose levels climb (cash is abundant), then our glycogen levels rise (checking account is stocked), a portion of dietary fat gets stored in fat tissue, and then the excess carbohydrates, sugar, fat, and protein go to the liver, where they are converted through lipogenesis into fat.

From the liver, fat molecules travel in the bloodstream and are deposited in our body cells, most obviously into our fat cells. Fat molecules repel water and pack together so efficiently that 40,000 calories weighs just ten pounds in our bodies. If we had to store the same amount of energy in glycogen or glucose, with water mixed in, we would weigh more than twice as much as we do. Thank nature for body fat.

You may be surprised to know that our active brains use as much energy as our muscles. The liver is a close second to the brain, with the heart, gastrointestinal system, and kidneys coming in close behind. Once the fatty acids get into the cells, chemical processes tear apart the carbon bonds. The breakdown of the fatty acids pro-duces chemical energy that our bodies can use. When glucose and glycogen stores are low, the body reaches for fat, its certificate of deposit, for energy.

When fat malfunctions, however, none of this happens. Instead, the fats and sugars we consume enter our bloodstream and, instead of being stored in fat tissue, go wandering through our circulatory system. They form deposits in places where fat shouldn't be, such as the heart, liver, and pockets between organs, impairing these organs' normal function. Ultimately, diabetes, heart disease, and liver dysfunction can result from malfunctioning fat.

When Christina developed lipodystrophy, she was unable to maintain an adequate level of fat, and thus unable to properly store fats and extra nutrients in her body. This resulted in deposits of fats in her liver and in pockets underneath her skin. Though dieters may dream of having no fat, the condition is catastrophic and potentially fatal.

A Solution for Christina

After four years of uncertainty, hopelessness, and endless blood-cleansing treatments, Christina's doctor told her family about a clinical trial to test an experimental treatment for lipodystrophy. It involved a newly discovered protein that emerged from a research laboratory at Rockefeller University. Receiving the treatment would certainly entail risk, because the protein hadn't been tested extensively in humans with lipodystrophy, and no one was sure what the side effects would be. But with the shadow of death hanging over Christina, she and her parents felt compelled to try it.

Christina, then seventeen years old, started a program of daily injections of this protein. For the first few days, not much happened. But by the tenth day, her appetite, which had been insatiable to this point, started to subside. She says, "I remember stopping to eat with my dad and not finishing my plate of food. I said, 'Oh my God, I'm full.' And that was the first day it truly kicked in."

Dr. Oral noticed medical differences, too. "In the beginning, Christina was still coming in weekly for plasmapheresis. Within a couple of weeks of treatment we could see it with our eyes—her plasma was coming out less milky than before. At the baseline, her blood was like cream, due to the abundance of triglycerides and cholesterol, but within weeks you could start to see through it. The moment we went to our planned final dose, her blood looked almost normal and the numbers were great. She never required another plasmapheresis."

As she ate less, Christina's circulating glucose and triglyceride levels reduced dramatically, leading to the remission of her diabetes. Fat deposits in her liver dissolved and its size reduced by 40 percent. The painful pockets of fat beneath her skin also went away. The experimental treatment enabled her body to metabolize glucose and fats more effectively, so that they no longer circulated in her bloodstream or collected in vital organs. Not only did Christina's health improve, but the child who was once slated for an early death went on to college, got a job, got married, and is living a fulfilling life.

The story of Christina and others with lipodystrophy offers a startling example of the importance that fat has in maintaining good health. Without it, other organs can't properly function. Strictly controlling intake and preventing excess fats in the blood could help manage the symptoms of lipodystrophy, though it would be virtually impossible to precisely match energy consumption and expenditure every minute of the day. But that's what life without fat would require us to do. Body fat allows us to absorb energy from food now and retrieve it as needed later, so that we can think of other things than eating.

We Have More Than One Type of Fat

Fat's responsibilities don't end with storing and managing energy. We also use it for producing heat, insulating our organs, and serving as a messenger to our immune system. Our fat plays different roles because our bodies contain more than one type. The type of fat that stores energy is called white fat, and white fat is what we want to lose when we're overweight. There is also brown fat, which is found in the neck, back, and heart regions. Its color comes from the high density of organelles called mitochondria.

The difference between these two types of fat is more than color. While the white kind stores energy, the brown kind actually burns energy for heat. Brown fat accomplishes this through a special protein called *thermogenin*. Infants have a higher proportion of brown fat than adults, although the latter have more beige fat. Beige fat was discovered in 2012 by Dr. Bruce Spiegelman, a researcher at the Joslin Diabetes Center in Boston. He found that during exercise our muscles produce a hormone called *irisin*, which sends a message to this beige fat and ultimately converts it to brown. It is not certain why the body grows more brown fat in response to exercise, but for the sake of weight loss, beige is the new brown!

The idea of manipulating white fat—injecting it with brown fat or converting it to beige—is now an active area of research for obesity treatment. In addition to exercise, exposure to cold has also been shown to increase activity of brown or beige fat in adults. Brown fat has potential to reduce white fat, scientists now believe.

Brown fat sounds like the holy grail of dieting—fat that burns energy so we can keep eating more. But even something this good can turn bad. Consider the unique case of Jocelyn Rhees.

Too Much of a Good Thing

Jocelyn Rhees was born eight weeks prematurely, with a birth weight of two pounds seven ounces. As with many premature babies, she was kept in the hospital for several weeks to allow her to gain weight and stabilize. When she reached almost four pounds, Jocelyn finally went home, and her parents cared for her as they did their three older, healthy kids. Though it is typical for newborns to gain about an ounce a day, by six months Jocelyn only weighed about six pounds.

Jocelyn's parents took her back to the hospital, where physicians ran a series of tests and increased her feeding. Nothing seemed to be wrong with Jocelyn, except that she couldn't gain weight even when eating ample calories. Her doctors referred Jocelyn's parents to a world expert on pediatric metabolism.

Dr. Khalid Hussain is a physician and professor of pediatric metabolic endocrinology at University College London. The institution is an international referral center, and he receives many patients with challenging metabolic disorders. Hussain is well known for treating and researching unusual types of low blood sugar and diabetes. In 2010, the young Jocelyn Rhees was brought to him.

Hussain did a number of metabolic and endocrine tests on Jocelyn to investigate her failure to thrive. Her blood sugar was low so he started her on continuous glucose infusion and increased caloric intake. Her insulin levels were low and her adrenaline, noradrenaline, cortisol, and growth hormone levels were fine. But when Hussain measured Jocelyn's resting energy expenditure, it was much higher than normal.

Unsure of what the problem might be, Hussain enlisted the help of other medical teams at the hospital. Geneticists tested for gene mutations associated with metabolic disturbances, the general pediatric group checked Jocelyn for unusual childhood diseases, the gastrointestinal team checked her digestive system. Tests were run for cystic fibrosis and infections. Every examination indicated that Jocelyn should be gaining weight normally. Feeling lost, Hussain also reached out to experts outside the hospital, but no one could say why a child who consumed six times as many calories as other children her age would not gain weight.

Hussain had been monitoring the child for a year, giving her continuous feeding and care, still she weighed only six pounds. Hussain recalls, "As a clinician I was very frustrated because I couldn't get a diagnosis. And for me it was also quite emotional because this child that had come to me wasn't gaining weight, despite everything we'd done. Not even after every clinician, every consultant who had an interest in weight gain had seen her. It was also frustrating for the family because they all wanted to go home, and I couldn't send her home because she needed IV glucose."

Finally, after a year of searching, a hint emerged. The doctor had ordered biopsies of Jocelyn's liver, muscle, and adipose tissue. Her liver and muscle biopsies were normal, but her adipose sample showed extraordinarily high amounts of brown fat. It was the first time during his entire investigation that he had found something insightful. "Excessive levels of brown fat would explain everything," Hussain says. "It seemed that the brown fat was burning the calories and the glucose was being sucked into oxidative phosphorylation and not being deposited into the tissues for storage." Indeed, Jocelyn's brown fat was shooting her metabolism through the roof, causing her to immediately utilize all the glucose she consumed. Brown fat also increases sensitivity to insulin, which explained her low level of the hormone. But too much brown fat was preventing Jocelyn from developing normally.

At three years old, Jocelyn still only weighed six pounds. Despite the involvement of doctors and scientists all over the world, no treatment was ever found for her condition. Six months after her third birthday, Jocelyn Rhees passed away.

Even something as beneficial as brown fat can harm us if it is out of proportion. Jocelyn's life is a reminder of the importance of having healthy, balanced body fat.

Fat Holds Us Together

Body fat's role is not confined solely to energy storage and heat. In 1899, Charles Ernest Overton discovered that the membrane around each body cell is made of fat and cholesterol—the two archnemeses of the modern diet. The membrane acts as a wall around the cell to confine the contents as well as give it structure. It is also a protective shield, allowing nutrients, hormones, and metabolic by-products in and out. In other words, every single cell in our bodies only exists thanks to the lipid-and-cholesterol membrane that surrounds it. Without fat, certain fat soluble vitamins, such as A, D, E, and K, would not be able to enter the cell wall, meaning we would never receive their benefit.

Brain cells are particularly dependent on fat. Parts of them are sheathed in a substance called myelin, which insulates them and ensures signals are not lost, similar to the way rubber insulates wires. Guess what myelin is made of—fat! Myelin is 80 percent lipids, which means fat is actually required to think.

Fat as a Messenger

Not only do we have different types of fat in our body, we also have different types of fat molecules. And some of these molecules can do fantastic things. A research team working under the premise that fat was useless discovered novel fat molecules accidentally.

In 1924, George Burr joined Herbert McLean Evans's lab at the

University of California at Berkeley. Evans, along with physician Katharine Scott Bishop, had recently discovered vitamin E and he tasked the newly hired Burr with understanding the vitamin's chemistry.

Burr got to work with his lab-technician wife, Mildred, to conduct experiments on rats and determine the nutritional role of vitamin E by omitting it from the rats' diet. But somehow, a lipid component containing vitamin E was still getting into the food. To prevent this, the Burrs removed all fats from the regimen. They fed the animals only sugar, casein (milk protein), vitamins, and some salt. Then the Burrs purified everything to remove even the slightest fat residue.

They expected to proceed with the experiment as planned, but soon a new problem developed. The rats became sick—their skin became scaly and full of dandruff, they lost fur around the face and throat, developed sores, and their tails and paws became inflamed. They continuously lost weight and, after three to four months, died. An examination afterward showed that the rats also had severe damage to their kidneys and urinary tracts.

The Burrs consulted nutrition experts to understand how to change the rats' diet to avoid this extreme reaction. Nutritionists in the 1920s and 1930s insisted that fat was not necessary for a healthy diet. The Burrs added nutritional supplements to the rats' feed but still they continued to die.

Having exhausted all possibilities, the Burrs tried adding some fat back into the diet. They started with just a few drops of lard a day. Soon, the rats' health began to improve. The inflammation subsided, and they stopped dying. To the Burrs it was clear that the common medical belief of the time—that fat was unimportant—was wrong. They were sure that fat was keeping the rats alive.

The Burrs set out to understand what exactly in the fat was saving the rats. After a year of experimentation, they identified the essential element in lard that prevented the rats from dying: linoleic acid.

Linoleic acid is a fatty acid, but its function is not to store calories. Instead, it is a signaling molecule that suppresses inflammation in the body. When linoleic acid was missing, the rats developed symptoms of inflammatory disease—the scaly skin, dandruff, inflammation, and sores. Replacing this fatty acid enabled signaling within the immune system to resume, reduced inflammation, and allowed the rats to live.

George Burr published these findings, but the bias against fat was so strong that he received a letter of condolence for concluding that dietary fat was important. Since the Burrs' experiments, however, other scientists have shown that linoleic acid gives rise to a number of fatty acids called eicosanoids. These are fat molecules in the body that derive from the lipids in the cell membrane. Instead of providing energy, however, they serve as short-distance messengers that can affect nearby organs and fat itself. Problems with this type of fatty acid have been linked not just to inflammation but also to cancer, arthritis, and other disorders.

One of the most studied groups of eicosanoids is prostaglandins, which are involved in sensitizing our bodies to pain. Prostaglandins also play a key role in pregnancy and are capable of inducing labor. Who'd have thought fat was so important for procreation?

Just like the scientists whom the Burrs consulted in the 1930s, people still assume that all fat is bad. But researchers from van Leeuwenhoek onward have showed us that fat is involved in the management of our energy stores, thermal regulation, keeping our cells intact, and, surprisingly, in sending signals within our bodies.

As profound as the early research on fat was between the discovery of the fat cell and the isolation of fatty acids, what researchers found in the 1970s through the 1990s was even more startling. Fat, it was revealed, could actually talk.

Chapter 2

Fat Can Talk

The Maliks were a close-knit Pakistani family that migrated to Britain in the late 1980s in search of better jobs and education. Many Pakistanis had made this same trip before them, and by this time were the second largest immigrant group in Britain. The Maliks settled down in the area of Luton, about an hour north of London, and quickly became part of their native community that sustained its culture from the homeland.

The Maliks were a consanguineous couple—married second cousins—common in certain parts of the world. They had three children, of whom Layla was the oldest. Born in 1989, weighing seven pounds, ten ounces, she seemed like a normal, healthy baby, actively exploring the world around her. However, as Layla grew into her first year, things started to change. She developed an enormous appetite and became obsessive about eating. She would finish a bowl of food and cry until she was given another. Her parents knew this was unusual, but suspected it was a temporary stage of development. As Layla continued to grow, however, so did her appetite, and before long she was obese.

The family tried to reduce her food intake by cutting calories and encouraging more activity, but it was to no avail. Layla responded with violent protests if she did not get as much to eat as she wanted. Tantrums, shouting, hitting, storming the cupboards became a regular part of the family's home life. And as her appetite increased, Layla became more inventive at finding food, burrowing through the trash and breaking into secured cabinets. Once she even forced open a locked freezer and ate frozen fish.

Layla's parents naturally grew alarmed at the actions of their once well-behaved child. Everyone else in the family had normal appetites and weight. Why was one child so completely different? As Layla started school, things became even more difficult. Given Layla's large and unusual appearance, she had trouble socializing. And adults in the community chided the family for not doing more to control her weight.

The parents consulted physicians and dieticians. The common advice was to provide nutritious foods lower in calories, and enforce exercise. The Maliks complied with the guidance, but limiting Layla's intake of food only served to increase her violent outbursts and desperate search for food.

The Maliks sought help from additional pediatricians and endocrinologists, who assessed Layla for various physical and mental-health problems. They tested her for a thyroid disorder, as low thyroid levels could lead to weight gain, but a blood test showed that her thyroid hormone levels were normal. They checked for Cushing's syndrome, a disorder caused by high levels of cortisol leading to fat deposits in the midsection, face, and back, but the tests showed that this wasn't a problem. They also tested Layla's pituitary and adrenal glands—impairments in either could cause slower metabolism and weight gain, but, once again, the levels were fine.

With hormones excluded as a cause of the problem, Layla's doctors evaluated her for genetic defects that can lead to obesity. They tested for Prader-Willi syndrome, a rare genetic disorder that causes obesity due to constant hunger: Layla lacked other symptoms of the disease such as narrowing of the forehead, learning disabilities, and speech problems. She was also tested for Bardet-Biedl and Alstrom's syndromes, genetic disorders that cause vision loss and diabetes as well as obesity. These tests came back negative.

No one was really sure of the root cause of Layla's ferocious drive to eat. Nothing seemed able to stop her. The doctors had run out of possible diagnoses and the Maliks had run out of options. Layla, it seemed, was destined for a lifetime of obesity.

The Findings in Fat Research

In the 1950s, two unlikely scientific developments significantly impacted the study of adipose. First, in 1950, a new research tool was introduced to science. It wasn't a microscope or lab technique, it was a mouse. A mouse with a genetic mutation that caused it to have severe obesity was now available to scientists. This creature, called *ob*,* changed the course of fat research. It had unstoppable eating behavior that caused it to weigh three times as much as a normal mouse and have five times as much fat, leading ultimately to diabetes. In this mouse, researchers had a living system of obesity on which to experiment.

The second development was an unforeseen leap in a different field of science. In 1957, the Soviet Union surprised the world with the launch of Sputnik, the first Earth satellite. This significant breakthrough precipitated a race for technological advancement. In reaction, the United States and other countries exponentially increased investment into scientific research. A portion of the increased funding was directed into the development of new scientific tools. Advances were made in biological separation techniques, such as gel electrophoresis and high pressure liquid chromatography. Both methods allowed the separation of cell components and the identification of cellular proteins. Now researchers had means other than a microscope with which to examine cell contents.

These tools, combined with the living system of the *ob* mouse, created many new research avenues. No longer confined to examining isolated cells under a microscope, researchers could now use the mouse to monitor the activity of living fat tissue and its impact on other organs. Scientists were able to more fully characterize enzymes in adipose tissue, the movement of proteins into and out of fat cells,

---

*The scientific name of the mice is *ob/ob*. Genetic nomenclature uses italics with the gene name given twice to denote that both copies of the gene have defects. For simplicity, the gene name is used only once in this book.

and gain a clearer understanding of fat metabolism. Suddenly, there was a lot of talk about fat. Scientific periodicals dedicated to the subject were established, such as *The Journal of Lipid Research*.

Although the understanding of fat was growing rapidly, the most astounding insights were yet to come. In a twenty-two-year period, from 1973 to 1995, two scientists from different countries, spanning different generations, revealed how little we actually knew about the organ we love to loathe.

Something in the Blood

The first breakthrough discovery came from The Jackson Laboratory in Bar Harbor, Maine. Jackson is a breeding ground, literally, for world-class animal models of disease. Hundreds of mouse breeds are created there to embody human disease states such as cancer, Alzheimer's, and diabetes. Scientists study these mice to gain deeper insight into diseases. The *ob* mouse that revolutionized fat research had first been identified at The Jackson Laboratory.

Douglas Coleman was a scientist at Jackson from 1958 to 1991. He had a friendly face, made larger by a receding hairline and oversized glasses. Coleman grew up in Canada and developed an early interest in science, eventually attending McMaster University. He went on to the University of Wisconsin, where he earned a PhD in biochemistry in 1958. He had planned to return to Canada after graduating, but the prospects for work there weren't promising. Instead he took a job at The Jackson Laboratory. His plan was to remain for only a year or two, but as Coleman, who died in 2014, recalled, "The laboratory provided a very fertile environment—with excellent colleagues and world-class mouse models of disease—and I spent my entire career in Bar Harbor. I never dreamed that I would work on obesity and diabetes. . . ."

One day in 1965 a researcher asked for Coleman's help to characterize a new strain of obese mice that had just been bred in the lab. These mice, called *db*, were different from the *ob* mice. Not only were they obese, but they had a more severe form of diabetes. Coleman studied the mice for weeks and developed a hunch: there must be something in the blood of the *db* mouse that was causing the disease to intensify. He arranged an experiment that would transfer the blood of a *db* mouse into an *ob* mouse to observe the changes that would result. Using a technique in physiology called parabiosis, he sutured together sections of the two animals' tissues that enabled their blood to be exchanged. If there was something in the blood of the *db* mouse causing severe diabetes, then the *ob* mouse should display the same symptoms.

After the delicate task of surgically preparing the mice, Coleman was looking forward to seeing the experiment's results. The outcome, however, was drastically different from what he had anticipated. Once the blood flows of the two mice were connected and the *ob* mouse received blood from *db*, *ob* did not develop the same symptoms as *db*. Its diabetes and obesity did not worsen, as Coleman had expected. Instead, the *ob* mouse grew *thin*. The mouse that had been three times the size of a normal specimen and couldn't stop gorging on food had now lost its appetite and refused to eat even as it was wasting away. The *ob* mouse had such a profound loss of appetite that it died of starvation.

Yet there was no change in the *db* mouse at all. Lack of appetite and thinness was not a trait either mouse exhibited before being sutured together, and now it seemed to appear out of nowhere in *ob*. Coleman then connected a normal mouse to the *db* mouse to see what would happen. Surprisingly, the normal animal also lost its appetite and died of starvation.

Fascinated, Coleman assessed this confounding new puzzle. There was something circulating in the *db* mouse's blood that could powerfully suppress appetite. That factor had caused the *ob* and normal mouse to refuse food but had no effect on *db*'s own appetite. The scientist hypothesized that the *db* mouse was obese because it couldn't respond to this circulating factor in its own blood, and the *ob* mouse was obese because it didn't make this circulating factor at all. Coleman was exhilarated as he recognized that this substance, whatever it was, could be a cure for obesity.

Into the Hospital

Layla's weight was approaching three times what was normal. All the medical guidance she received hadn't solved her problem. She'd gotten so heavy it became hard to walk. Her thighs rubbed together and chafed, and her doctors had to perform surgery on her legs to offset the damage caused by her overbearing weight. Liposuction was also performed to make it easier to move. This helped for a while, but Layla's unnatural appetite persisted, and her fat returned after just a few months.

Before long there was no more running in the schoolyard with her friends or cavorting in the house with her siblings. She was now unable to experience the normal life of a child. Layla felt miserable. Yet she could not stop eating.

Unsure what to do next, Layla's doctors suggested that she enter a hospital where her access to food could be tightly controlled. Layla was now seven years old and would have to live away from home. Her parents couldn't believe it had come to this.

Once she was in the hospital, the staff carefully apportioned and recorded Layla's food intake. They weighed her frequently and monitored her hormone levels and metabolic markers continuously. After several weeks, the physicians noticed her weight gain had slowed. This was a step in the right direction, they thought. But months went by, and though everyone expected to see weight loss, it never occurred. Six months after being admitted to the hospital, Layla was still getting fatter, just more slowly.

That Layla continued to gain weight in such a controlled environment defied scientific reason. Worse, the problem was spreading. Layla's two-year-old cousin was now also eating unstoppably and becoming obese. Something was plaguing the family that no one could understand.

Destined for Science

Coleman's 1973 *ob/db* findings alerted the research world that there was a mysterious circulating factor in blood that might inhibit appetite. Several labs set off on a race to find it. Being the first to identify the factor would be a huge scientific breakthrough that would bring accolades to a scientist. Coleman himself tried for years to isolate it from the *db* mouse's blood, but it was proving more challenging than he expected. As time went on, some even questioned whether this factor existed at all. A new generation of scientists specializing in molecular biology would be needed to solve the problem. Enter Jeffrey Friedman.

Friedman was destined for science, but didn't know it until his late twenties. Now in his sixties, Friedman stands well over six feet tall, with curly brown hair and wire-rimmed glasses. Given his stature, he was first drawn to sports. He says, "I was a pretty good basketball player. I could play basketball with some of the best. I was a pretty decent tennis player also. But I was a couple years younger than some of the kids in my grade, and matured physically late, so I wasn't making it on any varsity sports. But I spent as much time and effort doing sports than anything I can think of." It was an early sign of a deeply competitive nature that would be critical in his career.

In high school, Friedman's family encouraged him to go into medicine. He said, "My grandparents were all immigrants. Among Jewish immigrants there is an attraction to medicine because it is a respectable and safe way to make a living. My father was a doctor and I think there was always an expectation that I was going to be one too. . . . When it became apparent that I wasn't going anywhere as an athlete, my parents suggested that I apply to a six year medical program at Rensselaer Polytechnic Institute." According to Friedman, they saw medicine as his "destiny."

During medical school Friedman tried his hand at research, but his early attempts were not encouraging. He submitted a paper to the *Journal of Clinical Investigation* (JCI). One review was a rejection, but a long and solicitous one, explaining what the flaws were and how the paper could be better. The other review suggested this paper should not be published in the JCI or anywhere else. He recalls, "I'll never forget the reviews. To be honest, I thought at the time that publishing was a monumental intellectual achievement and I really had no expectation that I would ever write a scientific paper that would be published ever."

Friedman received his MD at the astonishing age of twenty-two, in 1976. He had a year before he was to enter his gastroenterology residency at Brigham and Women's Hospital in Boston, so he signed up for a research stint at Rockefeller University in New York City to fill the time. It was there that he met researcher Mary Jeanne Kreek, who introduced Friedman to the biochemical influences on behavior. He started assisting her with research on the effects of opiates on the brain. He says, "I was really fascinated that there are molecules in our brain that affect our behavior and our emotional state, that these weren't metaphysical processes, they were molecules that conveyed vectors of information. I really fell in love with doing research."

During that year, Friedman was introduced to another researcher, Dr. Bruce Schneider, who had been studying *ob* mice. Schneider helped Friedman realize that by studying this mouse they might identify molecules that control behavior. His excitement about the possibility led Friedman to a dilemma: stay in research or continue his physician training at the Brigham. Friedman's colleagues from medical school were already making a good living, while he was seriously considering going back to graduate school. Medicine would please his family but research had inspired a curiosity in him that he couldn't ignore.

Friedman decided to turn down the gastroenterology residency and instead entered Rockefeller University's PhD program in 1981. His father did not hide his displeasure. Friedman says, "I remember he derisively said, 'Oh great, now you'll get to be paid like a PhD.' He gave me a guilt trip about his dream to have me hang out a shingle with him. But it really wasn't my dream." For Friedman, it was not easy to give up a prestigious and well-paid career as a physician, along with a family legacy.

But at Rockefeller, everything started to align for Friedman. He began working with James Darnell, who was a leader in molecular biology, the study of how DNA turns into cellular components that affect our body. Friedman says, "I knew it was an upcoming field. It was a way to turn genes on and off and see how that affects cellular function. It was a time of great excitement and change in biology."

After Friedman earned his PhD in 1986, he prepared to start his own lab at Rockefeller. That is when he became curious about the missing factor that Coleman had identified over a decade before. Hypotheses about the missing factor had been debated by researchers, but so far little more was known. When Friedman called Coleman to see if he had had any luck, the older scientist acknowledged that he had all but given up. Coleman just didn't have the right tools to identify the missing factor in *ob,* and his search had led him nowhere. However, Friedman was sure there was an approach using molecular biology that could offer a new way to find the *ob* gene that would lead to the missing factor. He recalls, "Through 1984 to 1985 a plan was coming together in my head about how you might clone the *ob* gene, though I knew the project was going to be long term and risky."

In the world of science, Friedman was a smart, competitive upstart but he had not yet made a name for himself. Identifying the missing factor would be a way to change all that, and justify his career decision as well. Friedman says, "I was ambitious and wanted to be successful, and I knew that cloning *ob* would be a way to establish myself. Even more so, I was motivated by the intense curiosity about what this defective gene was. If you look carefully at these *ob* animals it's incredible that a single defective gene could lead an animal to eat voraciously and weigh three times their normal weight. The *ob* mouse was another instance where a molecule was controlling a behavior. It was pretty clear that whatever that gene was, it was going to be important."

In 1986, Friedman established his lab and team at Rockefeller and entered the race to find *ob.* If the *ob* gene could be located, scientists would be able to study what protein the gene made, and the effect it had on the body. The endeavor had enormous risks, however. In past cases, when researchers set out to identify a gene, they had the benefit of starting with the product it made—a protein—and working their way backward to finding the gene that created it. They did this by translating the codes of the protein that led them to the gene. In the case of *ob*, however, there was no protein to start from. The hypothesis was that a protein made by the *ob* gene was indeed the missing factor. The team had to start by finding the gene first, cloning it multiple times, and using those clones to determine which protein it was making. Then it would be a matter of figuring out if that protein was the missing factor, and finally understanding how a mutation in the gene could make a faulty protein that caused obesity. Just the first step alone, finding *ob* in a sea of tens of thousands of genes, was a daunting task.

To get a better idea of why finding a gene is such a difficult endeavor, we must understand what genes are made of—DNA (deoxyribonucleic acid). All the major instructions for creating and maintaining the human body are encoded in our DNA. DNA is an enormous molecule that is structured into a long double-stranded helix, connected by what looks like rungs of a ladder. Each rung is made of two connected subunits called bases, and each rung is called a "base pair." There are over three billion base pairs in human DNA. Because this DNA molecule is so large, the molecule twists, coils, and folds upon itself like a ball of string into structures called chromosomes. There are forty-six chromosomes in all, arranged in twenty-three pairs.

Each chromosome can be further subdivided into genes. Genes contain the DNA codes of each individual protein in the body that ultimately make up our organs and tissues. Proteins build cell structures and execute various functions within our body. Our chromosomes hold an estimated twenty thousand genes that code for about as many proteins. One way to imagine chromosomes and genes is to think of them as books in a library. The DNA is the library, the chromosomes are the bookshelves, and genes are the books, with each book holding the instructions for how to code a protein that has a function in our body.

Not all cells have the same proteins. Cells in your eye do not necessarily make the same proteins as cells in your bladder, which makes sense because the body parts have completely different functions. Each of our cells contains a copy of our DNA, and different genes are "expressed" (ultimately translated to proteins) by different cells, depending on the role of the cell. Once a gene for a protein is found, scientists can replicate the gene (clone it) and create the protein from it. Once enough protein is made, it can be tested in various ways to understand its function within the body.

The hunt to find the *ob* gene in the giant pool of DNA was like looking for a bottle cap at the bottom of the Pacific Ocean. Scientists knew it existed, but no one knew where. Investing years of a career searching for the gene was an all-or-nothing gamble—failure would lead to academic oblivion, but finding it would lead to fame and glory. To complicate matters further, the *ob* trait was recessive, meaning it skipped generations. So narrowing down the region of the chromosome where the gene resided would be even more difficult. Friedman's team, with the help of colleague Rudolph (Rudy) Leibel, would have to cross several generations of normal and obese mice to find it. This was going to take time and tenacity. It was not a job for the faint of heart.

Jeffrey Friedman's determination inspired the team to start the mission. The mice were mated, one pair at a time, allowing the researchers to look for traits that were inherited along with obesity. Traits that are inherited together are often found on genes in close proximity on the human genome. Using this approach was a way to home in on *ob*. Friedman and his colleagues bred 1,600 mice in all, continuously analyzing differences in their DNA patterns. He remembers, "It was unbelievably tedious and repetitive. The only thing that was interesting about it was the possibility that it could lead you to *ob*."

This stage alone—just cross breeding mice and analyzing their genes in order to get closer to *ob*—would take almost eight years.

Complicating matters, the DNA markers and guideposts Friedman was using to target *ob* were proving insufficient. He had to find new ways to narrow in on the gene. Friedman and his team heard about a technique called microdissection, which had only been used by a few researchers in the world at the time. It is a way of precisely cutting chromosomes to target a gene: cells are grown in a culture, swollen in saline solution, and then dropped onto a microscope slide from a height of a few feet. The impact of striking the slide bursts the cells, causing their chromosomes to spill out. The slide is turned upside down and placed in the microscope, so that the researcher can see the chromosomes in the hanging droplet. The chromosomes can then be excised with miniature cutting tools to separate out the gene of interest. It is a delicate and painstaking process.

Friedman remembers, "The first three years or so was nothing but excitement that you could actually do this. It seemed unimaginable before these days. When I went to medical school no one knew what the cystic fibrosis or muscular dystrophy gene were. These were being cloned now. The idea that you could find a mutant gene in this manner was just the most exciting thing imaginable. Then, over the years, it became clearer how much longer it was going to take and how uncertain it was." There was emerging competition in the field, and if someone else found the gene first, Friedman's investment could all be for nothing. He says, "I decided that I was just going to work as hard as I could. That way if it didn't work out, I was never going to have to ask myself the question about whether I could have done more."

Out of the Hospital

Layla was still gaining weight. But it was time for her to leave the hospital and return home. The remainder of her life was likely to be spent in a pitiful condition between the agony of extreme hunger and the shame of excessive fat, likely ending in an early death from complications of obesity.

A member of her medical team, Dr. Shehla Mohammed, a clinical geneticist, wanted to try one last approach. She had recently heard a talk by Dr. Stephen O'Rahilly, a professor of metabolic medicine at Addenbrooke's Hospital in Cambridge, England, who had successfully traced one patient's obesity to defects in the gene for the proconvertase-1 hormone. The patient had been obese since the age of two and no one could understand why, but O'Rahilly noticed that the genetic mutation prevented the patient's ability to make functional insulin.

O'Rahilly recounts, "We found that she had loads of abnormal levels of prohormones in her blood, precursors of normal hormones, but she wasn't processing them down to the regular hormones. But we did suggest that whatever was going on around here must be related to her obesity too. And that got me thinking, 'My God, if you've got an endocrine defect that can cause obesity, this means that human body weight is under biological control. And there are likely many others with severe obesity who have defects in those systems.' That opened my eyes and then I totally changed my mind about obesity. It was like a bulb going on in my head. The regulation of body fat stores is not simply down to voluntary control or social pressures."

O'Rahilly was quickly getting a reputation as an endocrinologist who had a new way of looking at obesity. He was also noted for his excellent problem-solving skills, seeing underlying causes of disease where others couldn't. Dr. Mohammed asked O'Rahilly if he would look at Layla's case records.

"We Did It"

Friedman kept pushing ahead. From 1986 to 1993 the team had focused on narrowing the location of the *ob* gene. However, they were still working in an area of 2.2 million DNA base pairs in length, which was much too large an area to simply pick out *ob*. Friedman had to get creative. He employed another tool—inserting the DNA fragment into artificial yeast strains engineered to carry mouse DNA. Such yeast cells were well characterized and using them allowed additional tests and dissection methods to be applied, which helped him narrow the area of *ob* down to a shorter region of 650,000 base pairs. Months went by. Friedman recalls, "It was an incredibly tense time. We were close but we still hadn't located it."

There was heavy competition from other scientists who were looking for the missing factor. Friedman had heard that there were labs in Seattle, Boston, and Japan, all pursuing *ob*, hoping to finish Coleman's search. Friedman was all too aware that being second in science does not bring awards. Growing increasingly conscious of his competition, he worked feverishly. He recalls, "I used to worry that one day I'm going to get a phone call that someone happened to find a gene, and 'sorry.' That happened to people. It was very risky and that's what would drive me nuts. It got to the point that every time I got a phone call from someone I wasn't expecting to hear from in the field of mouse genetics, I would wonder if they were calling to tell me that someone landed on *ob*."

Friedman and his team barreled ahead. He put his personal life on hold for years in search of *ob*: "I didn't have as much fun in this part of my life. I had already met the woman who is now my wife and the mother of my kids but I wasn't going to get married until this was resolved one way or another. I was pretty obsessed. In my head, I was never terribly far from the enterprise."

Then another obstacle emerged—money. Friedman had grants, but says, "It was made pretty clear to me that if we hadn't identified the gene by the next review it was unlikely I would be renewed." He was fighting the competition, fighting for budget, fighting to prove that he deserved a place in science. The pressure was on like never before, which only served to make him push harder. Taking his research to the next stage, he used a method called exon trapping, which helped him narrow the region of *ob* down to a few hundred base pairs. Now the *ob* gene was in reach. The excitement was building in the lab. It was as if the bottle cap they were searching for at the bottom of the Pacific Ocean was now within a football field.

As they were pursuing *ob* another startling discovery emerged— the area of DNA that expressed *ob* seemed to produce a protein that was uniquely made in fat cells. All of *ob*'s effect on the body, its impact on obesity, seemed to be coming from fat. This observation that the *ob* gene was expressed primarily in fat meant that fat was controlling fat. If this were true, it would turn the world of obesity research on its head. With this exciting possibility at hand, Friedman couldn't sleep. He was determined to find *ob*.

Friedman came into work on a Saturday evening in May 1994. His associate had been working to verify that *ob* was expressed in fat tissue, but she had taken the day off to go to a wedding. Friedman was unable to reach her and unable to wait. He dug through her materials and found all the components he needed to continue the experiments himself. He worked into the night, set up the final experiment to see if *ob* was active in fat, and then went home to sleep. But he couldn't. He was back in the lab at 5:30 a.m. the next day.

That Sunday morning it happened. Friedman realized that he had finally found the *ob* gene and the protein it was making. And that *ob* was being specifically activated in fat tissue. "I went to develop the film and the results of that film told me unequivocally that not only had we found the *ob* gene, but that Coleman's hypothesis was likely to be correct. I realized both of those things in a flash, and I got sort of weak-kneed. It was in a dark room, I slumped against the wall. I immediately called my girlfriend and said, 'We did it.' The gene was in the right region of the chromosome. Its expression was altered. And surprisingly, though it could have been expressed anywhere, it was expressed in fat. I have to tell you that was an unbelievable moment. In fact, it was the closest thing to a religious experience I've ever had."

What Friedman found was that the *ob* gene was indeed producing a protein that was made uniquely in fat tissue and nowhere else. If fat tissue had the normal *ob* gene that made the corresponding normal protein, mice were thin. But if fat tissue had the mutated *ob* gene, it caused a faulty protein which led to an unstoppable appetite and ultimately obesity. By producing a protein that was linked to appetite, fat revealed itself to be a clever, interactive organ that could control its own destiny. Friedman and his team were elated. Later that day, he went to a bar with some friends to celebrate. He told them, "I think this is going to be big."

It *was* going to be big, but Friedman wasn't finished yet. Now that he knew where the *ob* gene was, he was able to clone it and produce multiple copies. Doing so would allow him and his colleagues to create its corresponding protein in the lab. Once they had enough of the protein, they tested it in mice. They found that when the protein was injected into normal mice, the mice got thin. They didn't lose muscle or bone, just fat. When it was injected into *ob* mice (the same type of mouse that had starved to death when Coleman connected it to *db*), they also became thin. But when this protein was injected into *db* mice, it had no effect. Friedman replicated the findings of

Douglas Coleman from almost twenty years before and confirmed that he had indeed found the missing factor.

Friedman determined that the missing factor produced by the *ob* gene is a small protein that is secreted by fat and distributed by the bloodstream, like a hormone, throughout the body. This protein's job, when properly expressed, is to suppress appetite. But the *ob* mice contained a mutated gene that produced a defective version of the protein, so the animals never got the signal to stop eating. The *db* mice produced excess quantities of this protein, but for some reason they weren't able to respond to it, just as Coleman had predicted.

Friedman next extended these findings in humans. He identified the equivalent of the *ob* gene and missing factor that was observed in mice. He injected the human version of the missing factor into the *ob* mouse and, sure enough, it had the same weight-loss effect. He proposed that this small protein made by the *ob* gene be called "leptin," derived from the Greek root *leptos*, meaning thin.

Friedman's research was published in the journals *Nature* in 1994 and *Science* in 1995. The scientific community reacted with awe. How could fat, that inert, greasy tissue that was thought to be the bane of human health, actually have goals of its own and even be controlling our behavior?

Friedman explains, "I would say it was an incredibly magical experience. It was an elegant outcome in the following sense: nature has a very fundamental problem in terms of managing your nutritional state. You consume millions of calories per year. You have pounds of energy deposited as fat, and there was very good reason to believe that it had to be somehow regulated. So how does nature solve a problem of that magnitude, keeping an inventory of millions and millions of calories? And the answer that became evident in that moment is to make a hormone, leptin, that precisely reflects the total number of calories that are stored."

Friedman's publications incited a flurry of research activity to better understand the effects leptin had on the body. Studies by Friedman and others revealed that the amount of leptin released varies depending on the amount of fat tissue. Leptin travels from fat to the bloodstream and binds with the hypothalamus region of the brain, which is involved in regulating appetite. It is as if our brains ensure that fat is being fed and cared for before allowing us to stop eating. Researchers also determined that the *db* mouse had defective leptin receptors in its brain, which prevented the binding of leptin and explains why it didn't register the protein's existence. This is why injecting more leptin into *db* mice had no effect. The *ob* mouse, on the other hand, had normal leptin receptors in its brain but didn't make adequate amounts of functional leptin, so its receptors had nothing to respond to.

Friedman's discovery redefined fat and created a whole new field of study. No longer could fat be considered simply blubber; it was a verifiable endocrine organ with wide influence in our bodies. Through leptin, fat could *talk*. It could tell the brain to stop eating. And by refusing to deliver the message, fat could induce us to eat more.

Friedman says, "You get a certain result and it's beautiful. It's beautiful because on that piece of X-ray film is a representation that in some constructs could just look like a few blobs, but to me and ultimately to others it had unbelievable explanatory power for how nature has solved an incredible problem. In a way that's the essence of beauty. It's some representation that has deeper significance, an enduring significance."

Friedman's discovery also was a life-saver for people who suffered from lipodystrophy, in which fat cells simply atrophy and disappear. Because these people don't have fat, they produce no leptin, and so eat ceaselessly, like the young woman named Christina Vena, whose story is told in chapter 1. The painful, debilitating condition was incurable and led, in many instances, to early death. It was a medical mystery—until leptin was identified and used in a treatment that was also a cure. Indeed, leptin saved Christina's life.

The discovery of leptin was so important that in 2010 Friedman and Coleman received the Lasker Award for their discovery, one of the most prestigious accolades given for scientific research. Friedman had made his mark on science. And his father was proud.

A Cure for Layla

Dr. O'Rahilly had excitedly read about Friedman's discovery of the *ob* gene and its implications for obesity. When he assessed Layla's record, his hunch told him that she might have a genetic mutation in *ob*. She had many medical similarities to the *ob* mice—she was extraordinarily obese, had an unstoppable urge to eat, and also had high levels of insulin. Eager to test his hypothesis, O'Rahilly obtained a skin biopsy from Layla and asked his team to do genetic analysis to search for signs of mutation in *ob*. They used gel electrophoresis, a method in which the bands of genes are separated and can be differentiated based on their position in the gel. He had hoped the test would report back a mutation in the *ob* gene, but the test revealed that Layla didn't have the band where *ob* was to appear.

O'Rahilly was dejected. He had thought he might have found the first human example of the *ob* mutation. Even worse, he still didn't know the underlying cause of Layla's obesity. He remained puzzled at the reason behind her enormous appetite and unstoppable weight gain.

Several months later, a new clinical research fellow, Sadaf Farooqi, joined the lab. Her first project was to evaluate a new test that supposedly could measure leptin levels in blood. The assay seemed to work, so O'Rahilly asked her to test the blood samples of Layla and her obese cousin. Farooqi recalls, "I expected the blood of these children to have high levels of leptin because fat produces leptin and they were very heavy. Actually, when I tested them, they had undetectable levels of leptin. My first thought was 'I did the experiment wrong' because this was very unusual. We didn't have any more samples for a second test, so I tracked down the families to get more blood. When I tested them, again, I confirmed there was no leptin. I thought, 'Gosh I think there's something to this.'"

The team went back to look at Layla's DNA analysis done the year before, examining closely the placements of the bands on films. They noticed something odd—there was actually an additional band that hadn't been detected before because it was packed so tightly against another band. This newly identified band was the one representing the mutated *ob* gene, and just as in the *ob* mouse, it was present in both copies of the gene. O'Rahilly's original belief was correct. Layla was a human version of the *ob* mutation, with no leptin. Finally there was an explanation for why Layla could not stop eating.

There was an ongoing trial testing leptin injections in patients. O'Rahilly contacted the company, which had licensed leptin from Rockefeller University, and was able to get a supply of leptin to treat Layla. O'Rahilly and Farooqi started administering leptin daily to Layla and her enormous appetite decreased significantly. She would eat only a fraction of her meal, unthinkable just months ago. O'Rahilly recalls, "The response to leptin treatment was dramatic and miraculous. Within four days you could see the dramatic reduction in food intake and it stayed that way. She was eating a quarter compared to what she was normally eating. She went from being a completely focused eating machine into a normal kid."

Further research would show that leptin not only reduces appetite but is also involved in fat metabolism. Mice without leptin tend to move less and burn less fat, in addition to eating like gluttons. Without leptin, Layla ate all the time, yet was unable to burn fat normally, which is why her stay at the hospital, under restricted calories, only slowed her weight gain but did not lead to any loss.

After six months of leptin treatment, Layla had lost thirty-six pounds. Her risks for diabetes and heart disease fell to within normal range, and she was able to be active again. Thanks to a continuous supply of leptin, she was able to resume the life of a normal child.

O'Rahilly and Farooqi diagnosed Layla's obese young cousin as having an impaired *ob* gene as well. The family's consanguinity facilitated the inheritance of the mutated gene. Luckily, the cousin was diagnosed while still a toddler and treated with leptin, which allowed him to avoid the painful childhood Layla had endured.

Since treating Layla, O'Rahilly and Farooqi have identified around thirty children with mutations in *ob*. O'Rahilly says, "In other countries, many of these children have died in the first or second decade of life. This is not just a cosmetic problem—this is a lethal condition. The obesity is so severe the children are immune-compromised. They can't breathe properly because of the fat so they get chest infections."

O'Rahilly has become a proponent of understanding the underlying biological causes of obesity. He says, "People still have really difficult time getting their head around a gene that is causing obesity. It's a gene driving a behavior, and no matter how many times you say that, there's a huge number of people who find that very, very difficult to accept. I think human beings dislike the notion that we're not fully in control. The idea that there's some strange genetic variance in our brain driving us to put our hands in the cookie jar— many doctors have a difficult time accepting this."

Layla for one is deeply appreciative of Friedman's research. She continued to get leptin injections, which enabled her to maintain a normal weight and live a fulfilling life. She is now a college graduate, an attractive young woman who has started a career and is getting ready to be married soon.

Though the identification of leptin was a landmark discovery, it was just the start of uncovering fat's secret life. Since then, it's been revealed that fat has an even more expansive vocabulary. Researchers have identified additional hormones that are made and secreted specifically by fat. These include adiponectin, resistin, adipsin, retinol binding protein-4, adiponutrin, and visfatin. Each is being researched to more fully understand its role in the body. Adiponectin is the most characterized of these hormones and has been shown to be vital for healthy fat distribution. (It is described in more detail in chapter 4). Far from being useless excess, fat is proving itself to be a clever endocrine organ with many ways to communicate.

Chapter 3

Your Life Depends on Fat

Eventually, as we saw, the scientific community accepted that fat can communicate with other tissues, and that its ability to do so is necessary to human health. And there is even more to fat. It turns out that it enhances our brain size, strengthens our bones and immune system, helps wound healing, and can even prolong our lives. We are observing fat's influence in places we never thought possible.

For most of these surprising findings, we can thank a persistent group of scientists who followed the data, despite cynicism from their peers. In particular, we have one stubborn scientist to thank for showing us fat's role in fertility.

Fat Gives Us Life

Dr. Rose Frisch was a researcher at the Harvard School of Public Health for over forty-five years. She was a trailblazer in the academic world not only for being one of the first women in adipose research, but for taking risks and asking questions that others overlooked.

Frisch earned a PhD in genetics from the University of Wisconsin in 1943, where her thesis focused on human growth rates. But over time the study of genetics became more focused on detailed molecular studies, and Frisch was interested in broader issues. So she applied to the Harvard Center for Population Studies, which investigates demographic changes in populations and their impact on sociology and economics. She was so eager to join the center that she accepted an entry level job as a research assistant, paying only a few dollars per hour. Fortunately, her husband was a professor at MIT, enabling Frisch to follow her passion.

When she was awarded the prestigious John Simon Guggenheim Memorial Foundation fellowship in 1975, the Foundation inquired about her Harvard salary, and Frisch's answer caught them off guard. Thinking she misunderstood the question, they asked again, "Not your monthly salary, your annual salary." She replied, "That is my annual salary." The Center was finally shamed into giving her a raise.

At the Center, Frisch partnered with its director, Roger Revelle. One of her first research projects involved forecasting the food needs of the world's population. This necessitated determining the weights of citizens of developing nations and estimating their calorie requirements. Frisch undertook the tedious task of collecting thousands of pieces of information, and as she assembled the data, she noticed an unexpected pattern. The largest weight gain in girls seemed to occur immediately before menarche (the start of menstruation in puberty). This in itself was interesting, but even more peculiar was that the peak weight gain occurred at different ages depending on each girl's neighborhood. For example, Pakistani girls in urban areas had their peak weight gain at the age of twelve, followed soon after by menstruation. But girls in poor rural areas experienced their biggest weight gain and onset of puberty at fourteen—a two-year delay. Why would this be?

Previous studies had correlated height and puberty, but no one so far had tried to link it with weight. When Frisch asked scientists in the field why no studies had been performed, she was told that weight in women was not worth investigating—there was too much variation, and nothing to be gained by studying it. But Frisch was convinced that she was onto something and pursued the idea. Upon further analysis, she found that regardless of when females matured, they experienced the same average weight gain right before menarche, which took place at an average weight of 103 pounds. For some unknown reason, weight was critical to puberty.

Feeling confident about her findings, Frisch published her work with Revelle in 1970 in *Science*, the prestigious journal of the American Association for the Advancement of Science. She had uncovered an important link between women's health and fertility, but instead of a receptive embrace, the scientific community reacted with dismissiveness and disbelief. How could weight influence sexual maturation? Who was Rose Frisch anyway?

She felt the sting of rejection when she gave a lecture at a conference of pediatricians. At the close of her presentation, she was greeted with a deafening silence. After a few uncomfortable moments, someone from the audience finally spoke. "What is your background, Dr. Frisch?" It was not exactly a supportive question. "I have my doctoral degree in genetics," she replied. Then a question came about her collaborator: "And who is Roger Revelle?" She replied, "Oh, Roger is an oceanographer, and the director of the Population Center, where I work." Again, silence. When she gave a similar lecture to a group of distinguished economists responsible for the welfare of populations, she said they thought menarche was a type of vegetable!

Even among her colleagues at Harvard, Frisch struggled for acceptance. "Not only was it hard to be a woman in that role, but the subject matter she was talking about, sex and menarche and fertility, were things not many people discussed," Lisa Berkman, a director of the Population Center at Harvard, said about Frisch in the *New York Times*. "The men at the Pop Center would ask her to take notes as if she were a secretary, and there she was, equally strong as a scientist."

Not all reactions to her work were negative. Frisch had the support of an elite group of researchers in endocrinology and reproductive biology. She had the added advantage of stubbornness. Grace Wyshak, a biostatistician at the School of Public Health, was Frisch's close collaborator and friend. They worked on many studies together and supported each other in an environment that was not always welcoming of women or their issues. Wyshak says, "Rose stuck to her guns. She didn't say 'Well, they don't like my paper, I'm going to forget it.' She worked very hard to keep at it."

That tenacity kept Frisch digging for answers. She wanted to know which component of body weight enabled the onset of puberty. Was it water, muscle, soft tissue, bone, or fat? Frisch used various methods to determine body composition of girls, including water-weight estimates and eventually, magnetic imaging. After an extended period of analysis, she found that the tissue that increased most dramatically during puberty was fat. Girls experienced about a 120 percent jump in body fat just before menarche—thirteen pounds, on average. Frisch determined that there was a minimum requirement of 17 percent body fat in order for menstruation to begin at puberty, but 22 percent body fat was needed to continue regular menstruation as girls approached the age of sixteen. Without this proportion of fat, girls would not be ready to reproduce. It was an astounding finding. People thought puberty started when girls reached a certain age. Frisch had discovered that sexual maturity was instead linked directly to fat.

To Frisch, the "body fat connection" made sense. The survival of a newborn depends on its birth weight, which is correlated to a mother's weight before pregnancy as well as what she gains during gestation. Fat is a signal to the body that there is enough nourishment available for offspring to survive.

Frisch published "Menstrual cycles: Fatness as a Determinant of Minimum Weight for Height Necessary for their Maintenance or Onset" in *Science* in 1974. Again, the study was met with indifference. She taught a fertility class at Harvard Medical School where she described her discoveries on the importance of fat to the human body, expecting amazement, or at least curious questions from the future physicians. Instead, her students looked bored and impatient. They were too young—and too male—to appreciate it, she thought.

With time, however, word got out about Frisch's research, and she started receiving calls from fertility specialists confounded by their patients' inability to conceive. Physicians would tell her of their own observations about weight and development. In 1979, Frisch heard from Dr. Lawrence Vincent, a radiologist in New York City. He maintained an office near a ballet studio, where he regularly treated dancers for injured limbs. In the process, he was becoming concerned about their overall well-being. He said, "When dancers weigh in, the choreographer sits there and watches the scales. If a dancer gains weight, all hell breaks loose." Vincent said that he often passed dancers on his way to work. Of one in particular, he said, "I did not see a starry-eyed ballet student coming from her ballet class; I saw a pale, gaunt seventeen-year-old with dark circles under her eyes and a downcast gaze. Her unhealthy visage bore none of the physical exuberance and vitality usually associated with exercise. She looked terrible." It turned out that the young woman had eaten only an orange and a slice of mango that day and danced for seven hours. Vincent asked Frisch to collaborate on a study of ballet dancers.

Together, they organized a group of eighty-nine dancers of various ages and years of experience. They questioned the dancers and studied their medical charts, and noted that only 33 percent of them had regular menstrual cycles. Over 22 percent of the ballerinas had never menstruated at all, even though six of the group were older than eighteen. Thirty percent had irregular cycles, and another 15 percent hadn't menstruated for three months. The average age of menarche among the dancers was over one year later than that of the general population.

Interestingly, dancers would resume regular menstrual cycles (or begin them) if they stopped dancing due to an injury. But when they went back to dancing, menstruation would once more be interrupted. Further research showed that dancers who had regular cycles typically had 22 percent body fat (identical with Frisch's original finding for girls in their mid-teens), while those who menstruated irregularly had about 20 percent body fat. Dancers who didn't get their periods at all had body fat at 19 percent or below.

Encouraged by her findings (even though they held discouraging news about ballerina health!), Frisch decided to study other women engaged in extensive athletic workouts. She recruited twenty-one swimmers, seventeen runners, and ten nonathletic control subjects, and followed them through the training season. She found that the average age of menarche in athletes was 1.1 years later than for the general population. But there was a twist: if training started before menarche, the average age was delayed even further, to 15.1

years old—a 2.3-year delay compared to the general population, double the delay if the girls started training after menarche. Each year of vigorous training the subjects did before they started their periods delayed the onset of menstruation by five months.

Another surprise: though most of the athletes were trying to lose fat in their hips and thighs, they were actually losing it from their breasts.

According to Frisch's results, heavy exercise and low body fat were undoing puberty. Once the athletes in her study increased food intake, they resumed normal menstrual cycles, though some resumed more quickly than others depending on how long intensive training had delayed normal menstruation. Some athletes were able to turn their periods on and off with just a three-pound weight gain or loss.

Now with such precise data Frisch's studies started getting traction. The scientists and physicians who read her study started taking note. No one, it seemed, not even women's health experts, was aware that the reproductive cycle required body fat. In the years after her research was publicized, female athletes would routinely call Frisch seeking advice on how much weight they needed to gain in order to conceive. Frisch's son Henry said some of those women named their daughters Rose in honor of his mother.

Reproductive specialists estimate that about 12 percent of infertile women are athletes, and say they see menstruation problems most frequently in ballet dancers and long-distance runners. Some recent studies have shown that 27 percent of dancers and 44 percent of runners have irregular periods.

Sarah Joyce, a competitive long-distance runner from Indianapolis, provides a modern-day example of Frisch's findings. Joyce developed an enthusiasm for running early in life, and competed in marathons. At the peak of her training in 2009, she was five-foot-one, weighed eighty-five pounds, and had barely an ounce of body fat. She may have thought she was the picture of fitness and health until she tried to have children. She couldn't conceive, even though she was only in her twenties. Joyce's drive to be fit made her too lean to get pregnant. After getting treatment, and increasing her eating,

Joyce gave birth to a daughter. In hindsight, she told ABC News, "I may have been too intense and I think if I try again to have another baby, I will change my regimen." In reflection, "There should be a balance between eating healthy and continuing to exercise," Joyce said. "I have made a conscious effort to add more to my diet. Now, my husband says stop putting nuts and cheese on everything."

Why do women's bodies need fat for reproduction and the initiation of their monthly cycle? In the 1970s, doctors Pentti Siiteri from the University of California, San Francisco, and Paul MacDonald from University of Texas, Southwestern Medical Center, discovered that fat is a source of estrogen. The subcutaneous fat (fat directly under the skin) in a woman's body can convert male hormones, called androgens, into estrogen. Fat makes this conversion by means of an enzyme called aromatase. Young women make estrogen both in their ovaries and in their fat. (The latter is the primary source of the hormone in postmenopausal women.) However, younger women who are very lean make a weaker form of estrogen that does not prepare the uterus to host an embryo the way the hormone normally does. As one can imagine, these women also have challenges with lactation.

In 1995, Jeffrey Friedman's discovery of leptin (the satiation hormone described in Chapter 2) revealed another important aspect of fat's relationship to fertility. After reading Friedman's publication in *Science*, Frisch sent Friedman her articles regarding body fat and puberty. Friedman responded, "I thought you would be interested to know that you can make an infertile mouse fertile by injecting leptin." The protein was another missing link that explained why low fat impairs reproductive development. Soon after, Farid Chehab at the University of California at San Francisco reported in *Science* that when normal mice were injected with leptin, they matured earlier than those injected with a placebo. The tissues of their reproductive systems, including ovaries and uterus, developed faster than those of the control mice. Human studies also showed that leptin increases during the adolescent growth spurt in girls, and that it potentially activates gonadotropin-releasing hormone, which initiates the cascade of puberty. And if fat does not produce sufficient leptin to get it started, sexual maturation is delayed.

It is not just female reproductive systems that are affected by too little fat. In grown men, loss of libido is an early effect of inadequate caloric intake, and if weight loss continues, there's a decrease in prostate fluid. Eventually, sperm motility and longevity fall off. With acute weight loss, such as when body weight falls to 25 percent lower than normal, sperm production decreases.

Fat also plays a role in male development. A case in point is a twenty-two-year-old Turkish man who had a mutation in both copies of the leptin gene and thus very low levels of the fat-emitted hormone. As a result, he had low testosterone, no pubertal development, no facial or body hair, and underdeveloped penis and testes. His thirty-four-year-old female relative also had a mutation on both copies of the leptin gene, and as a result did not regularly menstruate.

Once both started receiving leptin injections, they resumed puberty even though both were now well into adulthood. The man experienced an increase in testosterone, greater muscle strength, more energy, and an increase in body hair. He even experienced growth of his penis and testicles. His female relative's periods normalized.

What scientists thought was most remarkable about this pair, however, was the profound change in behavior that leptin caused. Certainly their eating behavior changed as their severe hunger subsided. But leptin also caused a leap in their psychological maturity. Before treatment, this pair acted more childlike and docile. But after only two weeks of leptin injections, before any significant weight loss, their behavior changed to be more adult and assertive. Fat, through leptin, turns on the switch that allows our transition to adulthood, both physically and psychologically. If only our body-conscious teenagers, so eager to jump into adulthood, knew how important their fat was!

But beware, just as too little body fat can cause reproductive difficulty, so can too much. Obesity causes an improper ratio of androgen to estrogen in both sexes, leading to erectile dysfunction in men and menstrual irregularities in women. The abundance of estrogen, insulin, and leptin produced in obesity interferes with the intricate workings of the reproductive system. For nature, too little or too much fat is not welcome. A healthy amount indicates that conditions are right for children to be born.

David Hoffman is a reproductive health specialist in Florida who benefits every day from Frisch's findings and those of her fellow researchers. He works with athletes and ballerinas who have very low fat levels. He says, "Many of the problems we see with these patients are due to very little body fat. I have a whole battery of hormonal and other testing that I do. Ideally, I want to make sure that energy reserves are sufficient, and I try to get their BMI (body mass index) to be between 19 and 25. But realistically, some of these patients will never get there. So my goal is to try to get them to eat healthy and see if we can get their cycles back."

Dr. Shahin Ghadir, a fertility specialist in Los Angeles, says, "In Southern California we unfortunately see our fair share of people with eating disorders. Anorexia and bulimia are two of the causes that we see in patients who are underweight. For those patients in particular, their menstrual cycles just basically stop. . . . It has been shown again and again when these patients are able to gain body weight, and some fat on their body and their BMI goes up, that they are able to start ovulating on their own."

Hoffman adds, "Women who are too thin and even women who are too heavy have higher miscarriage rates. The amount of fat has to be within the right range. If you get too lean, you stop ovulating and it's hard to get pregnant if you're not ovulating. Some women have to cut back a little bit on exercise and dieting while they're trying to get pregnant. But if you get too heavy, say with a BMI greater than 34, fat tissue starts making too much estrogen. This creates irregular cycles and interrupts ovulation. It's not healthy to be obese and pregnant."

Fat is important for our health. Without it, there'd be no puberty, no sexual maturation, and no pregnancy. The right amount of fat is needed to propagate life.

Rose Frisch passed away in early 2015. After enduring decades of skepticism because of her gender and contrarian findings, her work is now considered foundational. These days, fertility clinics around the world routinely check weight and fat composition as a measure of their patients' readiness to reproduce.

Fat and Bone—One Strengthens the Other

Fat's production of estrogen isn't just important for puberty and sexual maturation, it is also important for our bones. Very low body fat causes low estrogen, which in turn causes weaker bones in both men and women. How can this be?

It may surprise you to learn that fat and bone share a common origin. They are both created from the same stem cells within the bone marrow. Stem cells are the multipotent cells in our bodies that develop into various cell types depending on the body's needs. The stem cell that eventually becomes a fat cell is also capable of turning into a bone cell. Fat and bone are like twins that come from the same birthplace. As such, they have a unique relationship to one another. They can even turn into one another when prompted—it's been shown in the laboratory that after differentiating into a fat cell, that same cell can be provoked to turn into a bone cell. It sounds like science fiction, but is true.

So what makes the stem cell in marrow turn into a bone or fat cell? It depends on the environment and the needs of the body. Researchers have known for some time that people who are heavier have stronger bones. One trigger thus appears to be weight. Being heavier seems to convert stem cells into new bone cells to fortify the skeleton. In fact, weight is a better predictor of bone mineral density (BMD), a measure of risk fracture, than age.

Estrogen also affects stem cell conversion to bone or fat. Insufficient fat not only leads to very low BMI, but also to insufficient estrogen; both conditions cause weak bones. In patients with anorexia nervosa, bone fracture becomes a serious risk. Though anorexics have little fat everywhere else, their bone marrow can be loaded with it. It appears that under anorexic conditions the body neglects its own skeleton in favor of fat, ordering stem cells in the marrow to convert themselves into adipocytes rather than into new bone cells. The bones, loaded with fat and weaker than normal, are more prone to fracture.

Postmenopausal women in particular rely on their fat to protect their bones. Not only does their weight trigger stem cell conversion to bone rather than fat, but as the ovaries stop producing estrogen, fat becomes the primary source. Aromatase, the enzyme in fat that converts androgens (male hormones) to estrogen, pumps up its activity with age. This makes postmenopausal women dependent on fat for both estrogen and strong bones.

Dr. Jonathan Tobias, a researcher at the University of Bristol, studied cortical bone mass (the hard outer layer of bones) in over four thousand boys and girls and found that fat was a major factor in bone development. He says, "Estrogen has an important effect on making bone. And so, if there is estrogen deficiency, it affects bone formation. Excessive reduction in fat mass could have adverse effects on the developing skeleton, particularly in girls, which could lead to an increased risk of osteoporosis in later life."

Fat influencing bone via estrogen and weight-bearing effect is not a one-way street. Bone also signals back to the body by producing a hormone called osteocalcin. Through a signaling cascade, this hormone induces the pancreas to release more insulin, which ultimately increases our fat. Therefore, bone and fat reinforce each other—bone increases fat and fat increases bone; a reciprocal agreement.

Brain Size and Fat

The other organ that is surprisingly affected by body fat is the brain. The fat in mice with *ob* mutation produces virtually no leptin, leading to reduced brain weight and volume. These mice even have a reduced number of neurons in vital brain areas, such as the cerebral cortex and hippocampus. Additionally, their brains suffer immature development compared to normal mice, and have a higher chance of degeneration. Remarkably, experiments have shown that daily injections of leptin for six weeks can restore the weight of *ob* mouse brains. Not only does their brain tissue grow back, but leptin also stimulates more activity than before.

Fat, through leptin, enhances the size and function of human brains as well. The brains of the Turkish family mentioned above were studied under MRI. During leptin replacement therapy, they started to grow brain tissue in the regions known as the hippocampus, cingulate gyrus, cerebellum, and inferior parietal lobule—areas that have been implicated in regulating hunger, satiation, memory, and learning.

Extreme starvation leading to drastic fat and leptin loss can reduce brain matter. Studies of anorexia nervosa patients upon autopsy show reduced brain weight, and MRI images of living sufferers reveal shrinkage of brain tissue. It's also been observed by researchers in London that low BMI (less than 20) in middle age caused a 34 percent higher risk for dementia later in life. Fat and our brains are indeed intertwined.

Still, don't get too fat and happy. Fat on either end of the spectrum is not good for your brain. Obesity, particularly the type including high visceral fat (fat under the stomach wall), has also been shown to atrophy one's brain. A study by Kaiser Permanente in California in 2008 followed 6,583 people for three decades. Those who had the most belly fat between the ages of forty and forty-five were almost three times more likely to have dementia in their seventies than those who were normal weight. Another study done by researchers of the Framingham Heart Study and other institutions showed that brain volume is affected too. They examined 733 individuals with high BMI and noticed decreased brain volume in those with high visceral fat. Damaging inflammatory signals emanating from belly fat and traveling throughout the body, as well as possible resistance to insulin and leptin, may be the cause. The right amount of fat in the right place helps maintain our brains.

Fat Protects Us

Fat is not only important for supporting other organs, but also for protecting us from illness and injury. Our immune system defends us against disease and injury by sending white blood cells, clotting agents, and repair proteins to the site of a wound or infection. To do that, our bodies undergo a near miraculous process in which they build vessels at the damaged location to ensure targeted delivery of these agents. The process of growing these tube-like structures is called angiogenesis, and its important link to fat was discovered—accidentally—by a scientist named Rocío Sierra-Honigmann.

Sierra-Honigmann was a young research associate at Yale University in 1996. Her husband was working at the Bayer Research Center in West Haven, Connecticut, where he was attempting to engineer cells in the lab to make the leptin receptor, the same receptor lacking in *db* mice. Sierra-Honigmann was helping him one afternoon. She wanted to verify that the cells her husband was making actually expressed the leptin receptor, so she used an antibody probe, which is a substance to test for the presence of the receptor. As a comparison, she would use endothelial cells (the kind that make up our veins) because they were thought not to contain the leptin receptor, which would serve as a negative control.

But to Sierra-Honigmann's surprise, the leptin receptors showed up in the endothelial cells. This meant leptin was somehow interacting with our blood vessels. Sierra-Honigmann recalls, "It kept me awake at night. If I were an endothelial cell, why would I want leptin receptors?" That question spurred a new research project for her at Yale.

Sierra-Honigmann sought the help of Guillermo García-Cardeña and Andreas Papapetropoulos, two fellow researchers who were studying angiogenesis. They took cultures of endothelial cells and added leptin to them. What they found was something that had never been seen before—the addition of leptin caused endothelial cells to arrange themselves in tubes that resembled blood vessels. These were the early stages of vessel formation, a crucial process through which we heal ourselves.

Angiogenesis was a hot area of research at this time. Judah Folkman at Harvard Medical School in Boston found in the 1970s that the process of spontaneous vein formation was a major contributor to the growth of malignant tumors. As tumors grow, they need to create their own blood supply in order to nourish themselves and keep growing. Cutting off this process was thought to be a way to curtail tumor growth and arrest the spread of cancer. Many labs were working to develop agents to stop angiogenesis.

Given the sheer number of angiogenesis studies going on at the time, lab protocols were well established to test for agents that either inhibit or promote vessel growth. The gold standard for testing was showing effective results on the corneas of living rats. When Sierra-Honigmann and her team tested leptin in rat corneas, they found that the hormone indeed caused the rapid formation of vessels. They reported their results in *Science* in 1998.

The research community reacted with surprise. Even Judah Folkman, the discoverer of angiogenesis, was amazed. "No one would have thought that leptin has anything to do with angiogenesis," he said. "This is a paper that is going to change people's thinking."

Sierra-Honigmann's next experiment was to test leptin's effect on the actual healing of wounds. She induced lesions on mice and treated some of the animals with an agent to block leptin from reaching the wound. In those mice, the wounds remained open and healed more slowly than those on the untreated mice. In other experiments, Sierra-Honigmann says, they showed that "a normal wound in a mouse heals in 5 to 7 days," however, with leptin treatment, "it is completely healed by day 3 or 4." Once alerted to her findings, other labs tested leptin on wounds, and had the same result. Indeed, wound healing is observed to be slower in individuals with anorexia nervosa, who have very low fat and leptin levels.

Sitting just under our skin, healing our wounds, and offering padding from injuries and falls, fat is in the front line of protecting our bodies from harm. But there are other ways that body fat offers security. Sadaf Farooqi, the endocrinologist and researcher at University of Cambridge who worked with Stephen O'Rahilly to treat Layla (discussed in chapter 2), has known many children with congenital leptin deficiency and studied their metabolism, growth, maturity, and overall health. Farooqi observed that these leptin-deficient children were not only obese, but are also more prone to upper-respiratory-tract infections than normal.

As Farooqi studied their biochemistry, she noticed that leptin-deficient children had reduced levels of some types of T-cells, key immune cells activated by pathogens. But as these children started leptin replacement therapy, their levels of T-cells and other immunity components normalized. By replenishing leptin, the children became less susceptible to respiratory infections.

It turns out that many of our immune cells have receptors for leptin, meaning they have sites on their surface that bind with the hormone. Once bound, leptin affects the signaling and subsequent behavior of those immune cells. People with very low body fat often have a compromised immune system. In developing nations, one way malnutrition facilitates the spread of infections is because low fat levels reduce the effectiveness of the immune system. Studies also show that patients with anorexia nervosa with extremely low fat have reduced immune function in their skin, an overall decrease in T-cells, as well as reductions in lymphocytes, another potent immune cell.

That fat enhances our immune system astounded the medical community. And the surprises don't stop there. In fact, in one area of health where we normally expect fat to cause illness, researchers have discovered the opposite is true.

The Obesity Paradox: Can Fat Help Us Live Longer?

Dr. Carl Lavie is a medical director of Cardiac Rehabilitation and Prevention at the John Ochsner Heart & Vascular Institute in New Orleans. He has been a cardiologist for decades with a thriving practice and research career. In the late 1990s, Lavie noticed that much of the research assessing oxygen consumption during cardiopulmonary stress testing—a tool used to assess exercise capacity and predict outcome in heart-failure patients—incorporated total body weight instead of using only lean body mass. Because fat does not contribute much to metabolism or the perfusion of oxygen in the body, Lavie became curious whether removing fat from the equation would increase the accuracy of the test. He designed a study of 225 patients and learned that, indeed, measuring only lean body mass enabled better prediction of survival after heart failure.

While examining this data, Lavie noticed something else. Those who had a higher body mass index, and higher fat, seemed to live longer after a cardiac event. This result defied the common thinking that heart-failure patients benefited from lower body fat. He studied more cases and confirmed a correlation between higher weights and better survival after heart failure. It was a startling discovery that went against scientific consensus.

Excitedly, Lavie and colleagues wrote an article and submitted it for publication. The first journal turned it down. Lavie was convinced that another journal would pick it up. He sent the article to a second major medical journal, but it got rejected again. He submitted it to two more journals, but neither would run the article. Lavie recalls, "We had a really tough time getting the work published. One reviewer basically said, 'This is the most stupid thing I've ever heard of.' The second reviewer was kinder but said, 'You had better go back and relook at your data because there appears to be a fatal flaw.' Basically, they were saying they couldn't believe it." The medical community couldn't accept that fat may have positive effects in heart patients.

But other physicians were discovering this peculiar positive correlation as well. Dr. Mercedes Carnethon at the Feinberg School of Medicine at Northwestern University examined data from 2,625 patients with diabetes and found that diabetics of normal weight had about twice the mortality risk of their overweight or obese counterparts with the disease. Dr. Jill Pell of the University of Glasgow and her team analyzed the data from 4,880 heart patients in the U.K. to assess their ability to recover after angioplasty (the procedure that uses a tiny balloon to open a blocked coronary artery). She found that overweight people had a higher five-year survival rate compared to normal-weight and underweight patients. Those who were underweight, surprisingly, had the worst outcomes. Pell told the Sunday *Times*, "People who do not have heart disease should be encouraged to achieve normal weight, since this will reduce their risk of heart disease. Among people who already have heart disease, being moderately overweight may not be a problem and may even be protective."

Katherine Flegal, an epidemiologist at the National Center for Health Statistics in Hyattsville, Maryland, analyzed ninety-seven studies that involved almost 3 million people to determine how weight was related to mortality. She found that over a given time people considered overweight by the body mass index (BMI 25 < 30) were 6 percent less likely to die than normal-weight individuals (BMI 18.5 < 25) of the same age, though obese subjects enjoyed no such benefit. So having an extra ten pounds may help you in the face of death brought on by disease.

Scientists and physicians call this the obesity paradox: while fat has been blamed for heart attack, stroke, diabetes, and a host of other serious illnesses, researchers are finding that low fat levels may make us even more vulnerable to disease and death. So, being slightly overweight may protect us against dying from the very diseases that fat is believed to cause. No wonder some scientists and experts had such trouble accepting Lavie's results; they confounded everything they'd been taught to believe.

But why would fat be beneficial in times of sickness? The theories are still evolving. One idea is that as a body becomes diseased, it has an increased need for energy. Fat may help sustain body functions during sickness and recovery. The other possibility has to do with the fact that not all fat is created equal. Visceral fat can become inflamed and lead to diabetes and other ailments, but subcutaneous fat provides cushion and energy in times of sickness. Other factors play an important role as well. Those who do aerobic exercise and strengthen the heart muscle generally have better outcomes after heart disease even if they are overweight. Exercise also helps reduce visceral fat, and redirect it to the periphery (see chapter 4). Apparently, it is healthier to be overweight and fit than simply to be thin.

Chapter 4

When Good Fat
Goes Bad

Kathy Maugh lay on the operating table waiting for her surgeon to arrive. He was twenty minutes late, which made her think back to her college days. When professors arrived late for class there was an informal rule—if they didn't show up within fifteen minutes, the students were allowed to leave. She wanted very much to leave the operating room now and cancel her gastric bypass surgery. All this waiting just made her anxious. Her heart was pounding. Why was this surgery even necessary? Up until her third child, she could eat anything and stay thin. She was "skinny-minny," as she calls it. Now she was sixty-five years old and one hundred pounds overweight. She had hypertension, high cholesterol, and type 2 diabetes. How did she get here?

Kathy looked back over the stages of her life. She had been thin as a child, eating snacks and sweets without worry. Through high school she was active and could eat as much as anyone and not gain weight. Life continued that way as she entered the University of California, Santa Barbara, from which she graduated with a master's degree in biochemistry. In graduate school she met and married a fellow student named Tom, and soon after they started a family. At age twenty-four, after having her first son, she quickly lost all her pregnancy weight and regained her svelte figure. She had her second son at twenty-six and again quickly dropped the baby weight. Walking miles with kids in the stroller certainly helped.

Kathy embraced her time as a stay-at-home mom. She took pride in making cupcakes, macaroni and cheese, and other comfort foods for her family. Food was love, and Kathy was terrific at doling out both. She ate her share of the big meals, too. But she was so active at the parks and pools with her children that she could still eat almost anything and stay thin. Once Tom bought her a box of Clark bars because he knew it was her favorite candy. Within a couple days she had consumed the entire box. She loved to bake and could eat nearly a whole pie at celebrations. Overeating was no problem; her thin figure was resilient. At thirty-one she gave birth to her third son. And again she was able to get her figure back, but she had to admit it was a little harder this time.

After her youngest started school, Kathy resumed work on her doctorate but before finishing left to take a full-time job as a genetic engineer. She had always been driven and it felt good to contribute to the world in a way that was different from diapers and spoon-feeding.

Soon, Kathy started taking on extra management responsibility at her company. Within a few years, she was on the fast track and moving through the ranks. Each advance required more commit-ment, more time, and more travel in addition to her roles as a parent and wife. This left less time for exercise and preparing healthy meals. She remembers, "I would be sending out e-mails at 2 or 3 a.m. I was traveling around the world and eating in restaurants. I would work through lunch and then get candy from the vending machine." And over time, Kathy started gaining weight. At first, it was just ten pounds. No big deal, she thought, a small price to pay to be able to have it all—a family and a career. But as time went on, ten pounds became fifty. And by her mid-forties, Kathy was seriously overweight and diagnosed with type 2 diabetes.

The disease was only in the beginning stages, so her physicians suggested that they watch it for the time being and urged her to eat healthier meals and lose weight. She tried. She attempted to pack her own lunches and exercise during the day. Given the pressures of her life, making the right lifestyle choices turned out to be more difficult than she imagined. Coming home hungry and having dinner, doing homework with the kids, and then sending e-mails until 2 a.m. left little time for exercise. And, given the stress she was under, Kathy didn't feel like eating lettuce at the end of the day. She wanted her comfort food.

Kathy's weight continued to rise and she started on diabetes medication. By the time she was in her sixties and ready to retire, she was one hundred pounds overweight. In addition to diabetes, she now had hypertension and high cholesterol. As time went on, her diabetes got worse and she developed neuropathy, an irreversible degeneration of nerve tissue that caused tingling and loss of feeling in her feet and was spreading to her hands. This impaired her ability to function normally. If she didn't reverse her diabetes soon, she could develop another complication of the disease—blindness.

How Excess Fat Can Harm Us

So how does eating candy bars and pie on holidays turn into diabetes, high blood pressure, and, ultimately, cardiovascular disease? How does our fat, which does so much good for our reproductive organs, bones, and brain, turn into something harmful?

In chapter 2 we saw how fat communicates by sending messengers such as leptin to direct activities in our bodies. It turns out that fat communicates not just with our brain but with our immune system as well. This relationship is useful when we get cuts, infections, and injuries because fat can recruit immune cells to help protect the body. But when fat activates the immune system on a chronic basis, it can lead to metabolic diseases such as diabetes.

It was not known that fat and the immune system communicate with each other until recently. Dr. Gökhan Hotamisligil was one of the first to find the connection. A physician from Turkey who was practicing pediatric neurology in the late 1980s, he became frustrated at the lack of treatment options for his patients who were suffering from cognitive issues, nerve problems, and brain tumors. He says, "I didn't feel like I could really help people. We didn't have tools to truly help. . . . I carried all the burden of the patients and their families with me. It was difficult to bear."

Hotamisligil began focusing on fat when a patient with Proteus syndrome was brought in to see him. Proteus is a very rare disease in which certain tissues such as bone, skin, or fat develop disproportionately to other tissues. The disease didn't fit into any one specialty, and because this patient had a fat mass growing close to her spine, she was referred to Hotamisligil.

Hotamisligil recalls, "This patient had local, benign fat tumors that kept growing. These lumps looked like normal growing fat, but were huge, becoming the size of a football. They could be surgically removed, but would grow right back." Patients with the disease could have drug treatment to slow the regrowth, but that was the best option that Hotamisligil could offer.

Beyond the agonizing frustration of being unable to help another patient, the experience intrigued Hotamisligil. What was fat exactly? If it could grow on its own, then it was surely more than just a storage bag for calories. This question ultimately led him to pursue a research program focused on adipose tissue, specifically on the connection between obesity and diabetes that was becoming apparent. At that time, he recalls, "no one was quite sure why obese people had a higher than average rate of diabetes." So Hotamisligil set up a lab to investigate the problem. His hypothesis was that since obesity involves the creation of fat cells, perhaps the fat itself contained something that interfered with insulin action and contributed to diabetes.

After years of comparing fat tissue from obese and lean animals, in 1993 Hotamisligil found something interesting: fat of obese animals contained an abundance of a very potent messaging molecule called tumor necrosis factor alpha (TNFα), which was known to activate the immune system. This was highly unexpected, particularly given that obese diabetics are usually prone to infection, and one would think that an increased presence of the immunity-related molecule would make them less susceptible.

Hotamisligil studied the activity of TNFα and the immune system on fat and metabolism and found that high levels of the molecule interfered with insulin signaling. This interference prevented cells from properly metabolizing sugars. Hotamisligil observed that the interference didn't just affect fat but also liver and muscle cells, making all three tissues resistant to insulin.

This discovery was big news. Fat was releasing a signaling molecule of the immune system that was impacting metabolism. Since insulin resistance was the predecessor of diabetes, Hotamisligil's research offered clear evidence of at least one way that obesity might cause diabetes—by increasing TNFα, which interfered with insulin signaling. Later research would show that not only does fat tissue contain TNFα, but that adipocytes can themselves synthesize and emit TNFα to communicate to other parts of the body, particularly the immune system, making this molecule another word in fat's vocabulary.

Hotamisligil's research inspired others to investigate new links between obesity and immunity. About ten years later, in 2003, Stuart Weisberg, Rudy Leibel and Anthony Ferrante at Columbia University found another connection. Ferrante recalls, "We were looking for genes and proteins that changed when people went from lean to obese." This was an unusual avenue of research because, as Ferrante explains, "people at the time thought that fat was inert, and it didn't change really very much."

Ferrante and the team discovered that fat was anything but inert. In the fat tissues of animals who had become obese they found an abundance of particular immune cells called macrophages, which are responsible for engulfing and neutralizing dangerous particles, usually viruses or bacteria parts. Incidentally, fat tissue of the obese contained very large amounts of these cells.

Ferrante says, "In my previous life as a graduate student, I had worked in a lab that focused on macrophages, and so when I was looking at this list of genes in fat tissue I immediately recognized that many of them were specific to macrophages. When we stained them I was totally blown away when we found, in lean animals, 5% of the cells in fat are macrophages, but in the most obese animals more than 50% are. And when you take into account the other immune cells present in the fat of the obese, well in excess of 50% of the cells are actually immune cells. There are very few organs where more than 50% of the cells are immune cells. A typical organ may have 5%." The news was so startling that the team had trouble getting the study published. Ferrante adds that the "reviewers thought we weren't really seeing immune cells and our immune cell analysis was flawed."

Why would immune components be disproportionately abundant in the fat tissue of the obese? One theory is that when we gain weight, our fat cells expand to hold additional fat molecules, leading to intense crowding in our fat tissue. This crowding induces stress on the cells. Also, blood supply and the flow of oxygen become inadequate for the growing fat tissue. In response to the stress, fat tissue sends out signals to the body, screaming, "Help me, I'm dying here!" These stress signals take the form of molecules called cytokines— $TNF\alpha$ is one.

The immune system interprets $TNF\alpha$ as a sign of danger and responds by directing even more of the immune system to fat tissue. For example, more macrophages will be sent to fat, which will engulf those fat cells that die due to the stress and lack of oxygen. It becomes a cycle: we eat too much, our fat cells grow until they are overcrowded, they send out messengers that summon more immune cells, and as we gain more fat, the crowding continues and the loop starts over again. This is why Ferrante and Hotamisligil saw so many more of these immune components in the fat tissue of the obese.

The large presence of immunity components in a tissue is known as "inflammation." When we have an infection, such as in cut skin, swelling and inflammation are useful because they increase the concentration of immune-system components to the site of injury to kill off harmful microbes. But in the case of crowded fat, the chronic immune-system activation disrupts fat's normal function. One key effect is that fat no longer responds well to insulin, as Hotamisligil found. This hormone, secreted by the pancreas, enables our cells to absorb sugars and fats from the blood and then burn them for energy. When cells respond poorly to insulin, our pancreas just produces more insulin—it "turns up the volume" in the hope that our cells will finally get the message. This leads to an escalating spiral of more insulin output by the pancreas, followed by more insulin resistance by cells.

Eventually, our cells stop responding to insulin entirely. This is a very bad outcome, because if our cells don't take sugars and fat from our blood, the sugars and fats will circulate endlessly, and start piling up in places where they don't belong, such as in arteries, the liver, and elsewhere. This leads to type 2 diabetes and high blood pressure, and if not corrected eventually to vein damage, neuropathy, blindness, and heart disease. Additionally, since cells can't internalize sugar and fats from our blood, they are starved of nutrients. This makes us hungrier, which in turn induces more eating, creating more fat, promoting the vicious cycle.

How to Heal Unhealthy Fat

One way to break the cycle is to alleviate crowded fat—which means losing some weight. This is not necessarily an easy task. Kathy Maugh's case was typical. She had a stressful job and long, sedentary hours. Time pressures led to fast food, and traveling compounded the situation. Not only did Kathy eat poorly and not exercise, but stress caused the release of cortisol, a hormone that promotes weight gain. No wonder Kathy piled on the pounds. Her fat cells crowded in her gut, and sent out an alarm signal activating the immune system. Several types of immune cells and cytokines infiltrated her fat, and she became resistant to insulin. The perpetual high levels of insulin led to insulin resistance, and ultimately progressed into diabetes, high blood pressure, and neuropathy. And now Kathy was at risk of going blind due to blood vessel damage in her retina.

Not all people who become heavy get the health issues that Kathy had. All fat is not created equal. In addition to high peripheral fat (in limbs and buttocks), she had a large amount of visceral fat—the type that is nestled against internal organs in the gut. Visceral fat tends to be much more metabolically active, meaning it emits more hormones and cytokines compared to subcutaneous fat. Excess visceral fat is the most dangerous kind of fat, and high levels of it correlate directly to diabetes, heart disease, high cholesterol, and even dementia.

Remarkably, there are people who are considered obese who appear to be perfectly healthy, and are not at risk for heart disease or diabetes. These individuals tend to have higher distribution of subcutaneous fat, rather than fat in the belly area. Perhaps the best example of this is one of the fattest populations on earth: sumo wrestlers.

Fat but Fit—The Life of a Sumo Wrestler

The goal of a sumo wrestling match is to knock the opponent off his feet. If any part of a wrestler's body (except his feet) touches the ground, he loses. Toppling your opponent takes strength as much as heft, and sumo wrestlers weigh two to three times as much as the average Japanese male.

Sumo wrestlers do intense physical training that lasts all day, from 5 a.m. to 10:30 at night. It includes a ritual called *shiko*, in which they stamp across the floor with wide leg motions to increase lower body strength; an exercise called *teppo*, in which they move a leg, an arm, and hands as if attacking an opponent; a stretching exercise called *matawari*, sitting on the ground with legs apart and chest touching the ground; and *butsukari-geiko*, in which they slam their bodies into each other. These exercises, along with plenty of grappling and sparring, build strength, balance, and endurance in the wrestlers.

This intense all-day training is accompanied by only two enormous meals—one at 11 a.m. and one in the evening. The meals include *chanko*, which usually consists of seafood stew, sashimi, Chinese foods, and deep-fried fare totaling 5,000–7,000 calories per day. The wrestlers nap after each meal, which is thought to help them pack on weight.

Sumo wrestlers weigh in the range of three hundred to four hundred pounds. Their bodies contain lots of muscle, but also an abundance of fat. By any standard, the sumo would be considered obese. And yet they don't suffer from afflictions normally associated with obesity. Their plasma glucose and triglyceride levels are normal. Even their cholesterol levels are low. How can they achieve this? The question puzzled doctors for years until Yuji Matsuzawa at the Osaka University Medical School in Japan uncovered the answer.

Matsuzawa and his team used computer tomography imaging to examine the fat deposits in sumo wrestlers. His study revealed that although the wrestlers have enormous bellies, most of their abdominal fat is stored immediately under the skin, and not behind the stomach wall within the gut or visceral area (which also contains the stomach, pancreas, liver, spleen, and intestines). In fact, Matsuzawa discovered that sumo wrestlers had about half of the visceral fat of regular people with visceral obesity, and hence enjoyed reduced risk for metabolic diseases.

However, when sumo wrestlers retire and start to consume processed foods and veer away from their exercise program, they almost immediately develop more visceral fat and the classic problems of obesity such as high levels of insulin, insulin resistance, and diabetes. Evidently, the sumo's physical exercise and diet low in sugar helps him to avoid visceral fat.

So how can strenuous activity prevent sumo wrestlers from getting obesity-related ailments? As Phil Scherer at the University of Texas found out, they can thank their fat.

Fat Just Keeps On Talking

While Jeffrey Friedman was working feverishly to discover leptin in the early 1990s (as described in chapter 2), Phil Scherer was also working to investigate proteins being made and secreted by fat. Scherer came to the Massachusetts Institute of Technology in 1992 after completing his PhD in biology at the University of Basel in Switzerland. Scherer says, in his slight Swiss accent, "I started out studying insulin's effect on fat. It was a big area of research at MIT, but then I realized that everyone at the time was studying insulin. It was a crowded space. I decided it didn't make sense to do what everyone else was doing. So I started looking at fat cells and what proteins they were making and secreting. It was a new field."

After years of painstakingly sorting through dozens of proteins made by fat, Scherer finally found one that was uniquely expressed in adipocytes and secreted to the body. At first, Scherer thought he might have found the elusive missing factor that Coleman and Friedman had been searching for (see chapter 2). But as Scherer investigated the newly identified protein, he realized that it was not leptin, but an additional hormone made by fat. This new hormone, which he called adiponectin, sensitizes the body's response to insulin, and guides glucose and fat molecules out of our bloodstream and into subcutaneous body fat, where they belong. Through adiponectin, it is as though fat is saying, "Fat molecule, please come home." This is important because an excess of circulating glucose and fats in the blood are precursors for diabetes and metabolic disease.

Scherer found that adiponectin also removes from circulation toxic lipids known as ceramides, which are byproducts generated by prolonged exposure to high-fat diets. Ceramides are elevated in people with diabetes, and contribute to insulin resistance, inflammation, and cell death. Indeed, a deficiency of adiponectin has been linked with type 2 diabetes, and obesity-related heart disease. So along with insulin, fat, through adiponectin, helps keep our blood clean.

Scherer has since experimented with mice that make an abundance of adiponectin and end up being fat but fit. He explains, "If you take up too much fat and calories into your system, the best way to cope with it is burning it off by exercise. If you can't do that, then it is best to store it in your adipose tissue. And if you don't do that appropriately, the fat will end up in the liver and in other tissues, and it's going to do a lot of damage there. So if you breed a mouse that chronically overexpresses adiponectin, it actually ends up being an extremely healthy mouse, but it's also an extremely fat mouse because it directs all these excess calories to the subcutaneous fat, and it does much less damage there than it would do elsewhere."

Scherer elaborates, "Adiponectin is the reason there are many metabolically healthy obese individuals. Not everybody with a BMI of 35 has type 2 diabetes. Those people who are overweight, in some instances even obese, but do not have type 2 diabetes, are the ones with the healthy, happy fat, and they have high adiponectin levels. If we keep our fat happy, it can be okay to expand it. Though, really, it is best to not have too much of it to begin with."

Exercise has been shown to increase adiponectin levels, and vigorous exercise, such as jogging twenty miles per week, or high-intensity training for three days or more per week reduces visceral fat. It is thought that the intense physical regimen of the sumo is what enables their fat to be stored in the periphery instead of in the visceral area. And when the sumo curtails this exercise regimen, unhealthy visceral fat quickly accumulates.

Between secreting leptin to assist bodily functions, and adiponectin to clean our blood, fat is a benevolent friend when it functions properly.

The Last Resort

Kathy's doctor prescribed metformin to get her diabetic symptoms under control. Metformin is a common treatment for diabetes that works by decreasing the amount of glucose in the body and increasing the body's response to insulin. The drug did not fully stabilize her disease, however, so she also began injecting insulin every day to help regulate her blood sugar. She additionally took medication for high blood pressure and cholesterol. However, Kathy was still at risk for developing other complications from the disease if she couldn't tackle her underlying problem—obesity.

Food was irresistible to Kathy. Every time she dieted, it was as if her fat could sense the restraint and thrust her brain into wanting food. Her many attempts ended in surrender and a return to eating what she loved.

In 2010, Kathy met Dr. Kai Nishi, the assistant director of the Cedars-Sinai Center for Minimally Invasive Weight Loss Surgery in Los Angeles. A young physician who found his passion in helping people lose weight and get control of their lives, Dr. Nishi started his career as a general surgeon working in the Emergency Room, but soon shifted his focus to bariatric surgery. He says, "With trauma, if somebody comes in with a bad car accident or a gunshot they're depressed that it happened to them. So even if you operate on them and you save their life, they're not really happy. But with bariatric surgery, I started following up on these patients six months out, a year out, and they would be in tears because they were just so happy about the improvement in their lifestyle. They would bring in pictures of what they looked like a year before, and you'd see what they look like now. They would tell me, 'I have a couple of young kids, and I could never take them to Disneyland because I couldn't walk with them. I couldn't go on a ride because I was too heavy.' I had a lot of people tell me that they couldn't fly in an airplane because they couldn't fit in the seat."

Obese people go through so much that the rest of us don't truly understand. And when a physician such as Dr. Nishi helps to remove that burden from them, and reintroduce them into society as a normal-sized person, they feel empowered again. For Dr. Nishi, it was amazing to see that every day. He says, "I knew bariatric surgery was definitely for me because I was making such a huge impact on people's lives."

As Kathy lay on the operating table waiting for Dr. Nishi, she asked herself one last time—did she really need this surgery? Was she truly unable to reduce her weight on her own? Her honest answer was, sadly, yes. Kathy had come to realize that despite all her impressive achievements, weight loss was an area where she could not succeed alone. For years she'd been reinforcing bad habits and now they were just too hard to break. Despite many attempts, she was never able to adequately bring down her weight.

Dr. Nishi finally arrived. He calmed Kathy and reassured her before the anesthesiologist took over and sedated her for the procedure. Dr. Nishi then performed the bariatric surgery, which involves reducing stomach size—making overeating more difficult—and reattaching the stomach in a position lower on the intestines, thereby shortening the digestive tract to prevent the body from absorbing as many calories. It is a surgery that is performed on hundreds of thousands of patients each year.

Kathy's recovery took two weeks, after which she felt her appetite go down immediately. At meals, she got full faster and ate less. She lost sixty pounds in the first six months, and thirty more by the first anniversary of the operation. She started exercising regularly and was more careful about her food choices. She felt that bariatric surgery gave her a tool to help her manage her weight. Kathy admits, though, "Bariatric surgery is not a magic pill. It is still possible to gain weight if you're not careful. The issue is, as you get further out from the surgery you can eat more. And food tastes really good. I still have to watch what I eat and exercise."

Kathy is now Spartan about her weight. She takes time to exercise each day and watches what she eats. She says, "I haven't had a Coke since before the surgery. I used to drink Coke continuously. I haven't had a candy bar, which is a big thing for me." Her discipline around food means that even if someone brings her a treat, like when her sister brings her famous cinnamon taffy, Kathy has to give it away. She has to think to herself that the taffy "is going to kill me," which is difficult, especially around family. Kathy says, "My message to people is that surgery is not going to be successful until you make the decision you are going to do something about your life. And you have to make a choice for a healthy lifestyle, including watching what you eat and exercising."

Dr. Nishi is all too aware that a healthy lifestyle has to go along with any weight-loss program, including bariatric surgery. His experience from performing such surgeries taught him that if people don't watch calories and stay healthy, the pounds find a way to return. Dr. Nishi offers a number of weekly programs to help patients keep the weight off, including hiring a chef to teach them how to cook healthy foods, and a therapist for behavior modification. He says, "If somebody has surgery, and then they disappear, and they don't follow up with you, the failure tends to be a bit higher. We meet with our patients every week . . . because that's the best way to insure that patients will keep their weight off—to keep them engaged. What we've learned is that if patients don't remain engaged, they will fail in general."

Dr. Michael Dansinger at Tufts University also runs a weight-loss clinic. He insists on seeing patients frequently. He says, "What makes the most difference is people checking in. In the beginning stages of a weight-loss program, we check in weekly. We weigh and measure patients, and go over their food log. What makes an impact is they feel they have to be accountable to someone they respect. It is a great motivator. Without it, weight gain can come back quickly."

The benefits of regular checkups can make medical weight-loss programs extremely valuable. Dr. Osama Hamdy, medical director of the Joslin Diabetes Center in Boston, explains, "In our program we have seen that just a 7 percent weight loss can improve insulin sensitivity by 57 percent. That is the equivalent of two medications for diabetes management at maximum dose. The 7 percent weight loss also dramatically improves endothelial function," which is important for proper vein and artery health and prevention of hypertension, diabetes, heart disease, and stroke. With regular weekly visits and continuous guidance on food and exercise, Hamdy says, "We have helped so many people get off of medications, many are able to cut them down by around 50–60 percent and around 14 percent are able to get off of their medications altogether."

Kathy Maugh had her surgery in 2009, and has stayed on Dr. Nishi's program continuously. The reward for her efforts has been monumental. A month into her weight loss, she no longer needed metformin, insulin, or any other diabetes medicine. The disease subsided and her body began responding to insulin again. She continued on her blood pressure medication for three months after the operation until one day, getting on an elevator, she felt dizzy. Her doctor ran some tests and saw that she had gotten lightheaded because her hypertension had gone away and the medicine sent her blood pressure *too* low. Kathy no longer needed her blood pressure medication or her cholesterol-lowering medication. This was great news.

Not only was her physical health returning to normal, but there were certain social benefits as well. Kathy says, "My husband used to say to me that I would be taken more seriously at work if I weren't as heavy as I was. And he was right. It's not only the perception you have of yourself that is affected when you are heavy, but the perception others have of you. The big improvement for me after I had the surgery is that I didn't have to ask for the seat-belt extender when I flew. That used to be so embarrassing because the airlines were never quiet about giving it to me. Preventing the need for an extender was a major motivation for me."

Dr. Nishi continues to meet with his patients weekly, even outside of the office when needed. He says, "Every Saturday, we get together at a local park, and we exercise with our patients. We walk with them on the track and they can ask us questions. And we don't get paid for any of it." This is much different from what Dr. Nishi experienced when he worked in a hospital: "When we were working for a hospital, we pitched that idea, and they said, 'You're crazy. How are we going to bill for that?" In his own practice, Dr. Nishi chose not to worry about the bureaucracy. "We're trying to help people here. So that's what we do. I go to the park. I bring my wife and my daughter and my daughter and my dog. I tell my patients to bring their families. We all get out there and walk with our patients. Sometimes we have twenty–thirty–fifty patients; it's a huge group. The patients love it because they can hang out with us. They can ask us all kinds of medical questions. They don't have to come into the office and they're not getting charged for it." Dr. Nishi makes sure he is there every week. Kathy does, too.

Chapter 5

How Fat Fights to Stay on You

"This Doctor Doesn't Know Shit!"

Sandra was a thin woman with a strong personality and dark, determined eyes. She had a toughness about her and felt comfortable confronting what didn't seem right. Now, her assertive personality was finding use as an advocate for her eight-year-old son. Randall had been a healthy baby boy of normal weight, and his toddler years were unremarkable. But as he advanced toward school age, he started gaining an excessive amount of weight. It was gradual at first, then with each passing year he grew heavier and heavier. Sandra couldn't understand it. Randall didn't seem to eat much more than other children. But now in third grade Randall had become obese and was entering a stage when childhood friends can become unkind.

At first, Sandra tried managing Randall's weight on her own. When that failed, she sought medical help. One expert after another gave her the same explanation: Randall's problem was his own doing. He must be overeating and not exercising enough. How else could he have gotten so heavy? But Sandra was convinced that something else was wrong. Her son was not merely putting on a few extra pounds but gaining an abundance of body fat. She was determined to find help.

It was a frustrating time for Sandra. In the 1970s, the treatment of the obese was blame-heavy—if people were fat, it was their own fault. And if they couldn't reduce their fat, it was their own failure. The understanding of weight and metabolism was rudimentary at the time, and the low-fat and high-carbohydrate diets being promoted didn't work for everyone.

Just as Sandra was growing weary of her search for answers, she heard about Rudy Leibel, the specialist in childhood obesity at Massachusetts General Hospital in Boston. He was not only a pediatrician, but an endocrinologist and metabolism expert. Sandra thought Leibel might offer one final chance to get the help she needed for Randall.

Leibel entered the field of childhood obesity accidentally. He had majored in premed and literature at Colgate University, and subsequently enrolled at Albert Einstein Medical College, where he read by chance about how the brain regulates food intake. He recalls, "I used to read parts of the physiology and neurophysiology textbooks that weren't assigned on energy metabolism. These were just side passages that we weren't obliged to understand." He didn't know at the time that this extracurricular reading would become the foundation of his future career. He received his MD degree in 1967 and pursued training in pediatric endocrinology at Massachusetts General Hospital.

Leibel recalls that the department head at Mass General "showed me the first *ob* mouse I ever laid eyes on and told me that they were a mystery in terms of why they got so obese." Leibel took particular interest in these mice, which piqued the same interest that his extracurricular college reading did years before.

As Leibel advanced at Mass General, he also joined the faculty at Harvard Medical School, where a fourth-year medical student asked him to supervise his thesis on body weight regulation. Once he got involved, he says, "I decided then that it was the area I was interested in. And then the word got out and people began sending me patients who were obese because nobody really knew what to do with these kids. Everybody thought they might have some primary endocrine disturbance like hypothyroidism or excessive glucocorticoid activity, and of course, the vast majority of them never did. I started to see a lot of obese kids."

It was on a cold evening in 1977 that Sandra pulled Randall from his home and made her way across Boston to Mass General, hoping

Rudy Leibel would at last give her insight into Randall's condition. She waited as Leibel assessed her son for disorders that cause weight gain. Leibel took a history of the boy. Obese children were commonly tested for hypothyroid condition, and for Cushing's disease, an excess production of glucocorticoid. Leibel says, "This boy clearly didn't have any of that. He was just very obese for reasons that I didn't understand, and neither did anyone else." From what Leibel knew, the boy was not eating enormous portions of food, or sitting on the couch all day. Nothing he was doing seemed to add up to obesity. Leibel recalls, "I wasn't sure why this kid was as obese as he was, but this was an area where I didn't think it was his fault. I just didn't know what the problem was."

After some moments of silence, he turned to Sandra and said, "This is a mystery." A pause followed. He broke the awkward silence by giving her a talk about watching Randall's diet and making sure he exercised, and emphasized the importance of nutrition.

Believing he had given his best medical assessment, Leibel expected the mother to respectfully note his advice. Instead, Sandra angrily grabbed her son and said, "Randall, let's get out of here. This doctor doesn't know shit!"

Leibel remembers feeling waves of emotion at that moment. At first he was stunned, then insulted, and finally embarrassed as Sandra stormed out of his office, taking Randall by the arm. However, as he reflected on the encounter, he realized that Sandra was right. "I decided right at that moment what Randall's mother told me pretty much summarized the level of my knowledge about this [obesity]," he said. "I wasn't totally guilty because I wasn't any different than anyone else." No one at the time really understood obesity, but for Leibel, this was a seminal event: "I decided that I was going to get laboratory training. I hadn't really done any bench work at all at this point. But I decided I was going to go back and really train myself to do basic research."

From that inauspicious beginning, Leibel would go on to make discoveries that would completely transform our understanding of fat and topple the dogma that the persistence of obesity is simply due to gluttony.

But it took time.

Rudy Leibel knew where he would start his inquiry. Some years before, at a pediatric conference, he had met Jules Hirsch, who ran the obesity department at Rockefeller University in New York City. Rockefeller was one of the leading obesity-research centers in the world and Hirsch was a veteran scientist who at the time was studying changes to fat cells after weight loss. Hirsch had noted Leibel's strong interest in obesity, and when the Boston doctor decided to switch to research, Hirsch invited him to join the team at Rockefeller.

Rockefeller is a prestigious institution, and getting a position there is a significant achievement for any scientist. Most who join the faculty have extensive graduate and postgraduate training; usually they transition without incident. But Leibel's adjustment to the research world was not easy. As a faculty member of Harvard Medical School and a physician at Mass General, he enjoyed a generous salary and a comfortable lifestyle, residing in a large Victorian house in the tony section of Brookline. Starting over in research meant a huge cut in pay. He would have to move his wife and their two children out of their beautiful home, sell most of their possessions, and move into a 1,200-square-foot apartment at Rockefeller's faculty house. Says Leibel, "I went from Boston to Rockefeller University, essentially as a postdoctoral fellow. I moved backwards in my career. But I did that in order to be able to have access to a laboratory and time to train myself to do research." Luckily for Leibel, his wife was agreeable. "She said, 'If this is what you have to do, I'll do it.' . . . She never accused me of being out of my mind. . . . She was just amazingly supportive.'"

Though it was not obvious at the time, joining Hirsch and other scientists at Rockefeller in 1978 was the first step in what would become a distinguished career. With the memory of Randall as an inspiration, Leibel started with the basic molecular aspects of obesity, looking at how by-products of fat metabolism affect hunger and weight loss. He investigated genetics and hormones in obesity, and observed that some hormones, such as adrenaline, facilitate fat breakdown while others, such as insulin, inhibit it. He also researched the *ob* gene and the effect it had on fat.

However, with each incremental discovery, Leibel started to notice something unusual. Fat, it seemed, had an uncanny, sneaky ability to control its own fate. The first hint of its insidious personality came in 1983. Leibel noticed that when obese people fought fat, it had a number of weapons at its disposal to fight back.

Leibel and Hirsch had examined the charts of patients who were admitted into obesity studies at Rockefeller University Hospital between 1965 and 1979. In reviewing the data, they compared the food intake of twenty-six obese patients before and after they lost an average of 115 pounds. Although this was a significant amount of weight loss, these patients were still overweight and were termed "reduced-obese." This group required 28 percent fewer calories to maintain their reduced weight, which seemed understandable: when people reduce their weight they need fewer calories. But something interesting emerged when the scientists compared the food intake of the reduced-obese to that of control subjects who were never obese to begin with. The reduced-obese were eating slightly *fewer* calories than the never-obese group, but their weight was still 60 percent *higher*. Somehow, the remaining body fat of the reduced-obese was able to survive on fewer calories than before, as if it had found another means to thrive.

Leibel was fascinated. How could obese people eat significantly less than those of healthy weight and still maintain their excessive body fat? He teamed up with Dr. Michael Rosenbaum in 1985. Rosenbaum was completing a fellowship in pediatric endocrinology at the neighboring New York Presbyterian Hospital. He shared Leibel's love of literature, and somewhere between discussing Emily Dickinson and the causes of obesity the two forged a strong collaboration. Rosenbaum, who stands tall at six feet two inches and has long, wavy hair, recalls, "Rudy and Jules had all the qualities of great scientists and teachers. They presented their research clearly and in a way that was so exciting and enthusiastic that you just wanted to be a part of it." Rosenbaum went to Rockefeller University in 1988 and with Leibel studied the differences in metabolism in lean and obese individuals. It would lead to some of our most important insights into obesity.

Leibel and Rosenbaum recruited subjects to research by running ads. The requirements for entering the study were being at their highest lifetime weight for at least the past six months, agreeing to lose 10 percent of it on the study, and having their body's reaction to weight loss examined. For comparison, the researchers also recruited lean subjects who would undergo the same procedure. All participants agreed to reside for at least six months in the hospital, where their diet and exercise would be tightly controlled. It was a big commitment, but plenty of people were willing to be studied for the promise of losing weight. Over the course of the study more than 150 people enrolled.

The research subjects were allowed only a liquid diet consisting of shakes with a meticulously measured balance of carbohydrates, fats, and protein. The food was not tasty, but the participants honored their commitment. After an initial period of testing and weight stabilization, their shakes were reduced to 800 calories per day until they lost 10 percent of their body weight, which usually took thirty-five to sixty days. All during the study, participants engaged in physical exercise to maintain their usual levels of fitness. It was an intense experience, sometimes difficult because of the hunger and monotony, but they lost weight.

Once the subjects had been stabilized at their reduced weight, Leibel and Rosenbaum got to work assessing their metabolic changes. They found that after losing 10 percent of their body weight, both lean and obese individuals needed about 22 percent fewer calories to maintain their lower weight compared to someone who was "naturally" at that weight to begin with. This meant that most people who had lost only 10 percent of their weight would have to eat about 250–400 fewer calories per day or exercise that much more if they wanted to keep it off compared to someone who was at that weight without dieting. So gaining weight and then losing it levied a caloric "penalty."

How could fat sustain itself on fewer calories? In order to understand this, the researchers studied how energy usage in the body changed after it lost fat. Through complicated calculations, the team isolated the total energy expenditure of the body into its components, which include the energy used while at rest as well as the energy burned while active, such as during exercise.

Leibel and Rosenbaum noticed that after a 10 percent weight loss, the energy expended at rest decreased by about 15 percent. However, the energy expended during physical activity decreased even more—by 25 percent. So once we lose weight, our bodies are more efficient and conserve energy at rest, and are even better at doing so during exercise. Put another way, a person who has lost weight has to run five miles for every four miles a person who is naturally at that weight does in order to burn as many calories. If the dieter who's achieved a new lower weight eats and exercises like a person naturally at the same weight, the dieter will put on pounds. It's unfair. But after the hard work of shedding fat we have to work harder than those who have not dieted to keep it off, and are forever at higher risk of getting it back. So, even a temporary weight gain can have lifelong consequences.

Why would bodies of equal fat and mass require different amounts of calories depending on whether one dieted or not to achieve that target weight? Leibel and Rosenbaum hypothesized that changes to hormones were involved. They tested this hypothesis by drawing blood of participants before and after they reduced weight and found that leptin levels decreased significantly after weight loss. This was not surprising, considering that fat secretes leptin, and these subjects now had less fat. But in addition to lower leptin, thyroid hormones decreased significantly as well. Thyroid hormones regulate metabolism—when their level decreases, so does our metabolic rate. The researchers also measured adrenaline and noradrenaline, hormones that increase metabolic rates. When participants lost weight, those levels also dropped, thereby slowing metabolism. After losing weight, the body was making a coordinated effort to return to its known and comfortable weight by decreasing how many calories it burned.

Leibel explains, "Anyone who's reduced weight by diet or any other means, tends to regain the weight with very high accuracy. People will generally go back to the weight that they started at, not one that's way below or way above, as if the body were somehow able to sense where its normal amount of body fat is."

The decreasing hormone levels provided a reason why metabolism slowed, and why we expend less energy after weight loss than before. But the question remained: why does losing fat affect those hormones and change metabolism? Many labs had studied this very question; what they determined was that fat, by means of the leptin it releases, has the potential to alter the activity of our hormones and nervous system. Leptin secreted into our circulatory system ultimately reaches our brain and endocrine glands. It enhances the secretion of key thyroid hormones, and also noradrenaline and adrenalin, all of which increase our metabolism. When leptin is at its normal level, these hormones are also at their normal levels, and so is our metabolism. When we lose fat, however, and our leptin levels fall, the release of these hormones is diminished, and so is our metabolism.

Furthermore, when there is a lack of leptin, skeletal muscles become more efficient and consume less energy. This is mediated by a number of factors, including the decrease in thyroid hormone. Again, this effect lowers metabolism and offsets the calorie-burning effects of exercise. And this slowdown occurs whether one loses fat by restricting calories or increasing exercise. So through leptin, fat exerts powerful influence and can control its own fate by slowing down calorie usage.

Rosenbaum says, "There is a bias in society. People think that someone who is naturally slender but cannot keep a small amount of weight off simply has a slow metabolism, but someone who is obese and can't sustain a large degree of weight loss is lazy, slothful, and gluttonous. But there are many reasons that fat persists. Ideally, intervention needs to happen before obesity develops."

Leibel and Rosenbaum were uncovering the reasons our metabolism is slower both during and after losing weight. Much of it had to do with reducing fat and leptin levels. But there were still more mysteries to unravel. If the body was using less energy after weight loss, then people should also have decreased appetite, right?

Unfortunately, no. The reduced-obese craved food like never before. Leibel and Rosenbaum teamed up with Joy Hirsch, director of the program for Imaging and Cognitive Sciences at Columbia

University. Hirsch is an expert in fMRI (functional magnetic resonance imaging), which allows us to monitor brain activity while people perform various tasks. The team examined fMRI brain scans of the reduced-obese as they looked at images of food. People who had lost 10 percent of their body weight had much higher responses to food cues than those who hadn't lost any weight at all. When the former were shown pictures of food, the part of the brain involved in emotional or sensory reactions lit up brightly, much more so than those of people who had lost no weight. At the same time, the part of the brain involved in control of food intake had significantly diminished responses. So, losing weight makes us more responsive to food and less able to control our intake—a killer combination.

The fMRI observations bore out in real life settings too. When the reduced-obese group sat down to have a meal, they rated themselves as hungrier at the start of it and less satiated at the end of it than they did before losing weight. These perceptions persisted even though the amount of food was the same or higher than before they lost weight.

Leibel says, "We've studied patients as long as five or six years after weight loss, and they have exactly the same lowering of energy expenditure and increased drive to eat. We don't think it ever goes away." This is hard news for dieters and underscores the importance of preventing excessive fat gain in the first place.

Years after that fateful encounter with Randall and his mother, Rudy Leibel was uncovering many possible answers to the boy's weight problem. Through its most powerful messenger, leptin, fat can influence our appetites. It can cause our muscles to reduce their energy usage. It can alter our sympathetic nervous system, and control the flow of hormones such as thyroid, adrenaline, and noradrenaline. Most profoundly, it can influence our thoughts and elicit stronger responses to food, lower our inhibition to eating, and cause us to misjudge how much we've eaten. Fat, it turns out, is capable of mind control!

Though he never got the chance to follow up with the young patient, Leibel considers Randall's case a turning point in his career. It provided him with that burning question researchers need to dedicate their lives to science, and the outcome has been rewarding to both Leibel and the field of obesity research.

Many of Leibel's recent studies show that the body's coordinated response to enable weight regain can be reversed by administering additional leptin to those who have lost weight. His approach treats those who have lost weight as being leptin deficient, just like Layla Malik (discussed in chapter 2). Injecting leptin doesn't affect those with normal levels of the hormone, but it is effective in those who have abnormally low levels, whether from weight loss or genetic causes. Leibel has seen strong results in the early experiments. When study participants who lost 10 percent of their weight received daily leptin injections, they were able to control appetite better, their metabolism improved, and it became easier to maintain weight loss. Using leptin in this way is still experimental, and has not been approved for broader use. But Leibel continues searching for additional approaches as well. He says that in the end he is still looking for ways to help Randall.

Confirmation from Melbourne

Leibel and Rosenbaum made great advances in understanding fat and the widespread power it has over us. Meanwhile, ten thousand miles away, in Melbourne, Australia, Dr. Joseph Proietto was conducting his own investigations into fat's persistence. Proietto, an endocrinologist by training, has been studying and treating weight problems for decades. He founded the obesity clinic at the Austin Hospital in Melbourne. Over the years, he's seen patient after patient lose and then regain their fat. The cycle is debilitating, physically and emotionally. Proietto says, "You have no idea how frustrating treating obesity is. I had all of these people that came to me in the clinic, who were motivated to lose weight—clearly motivated. They would successfully lose weight, and then gradually they would regain. And I thought it can't be just that people are weak. It's got to be more to it than that." Proietto's frustration led him to pursue the testing of additional hormonal responses to weight loss in the hope of helping his patients keep off the weight they worked so hard to lose.

In 2009, Proietto assembled fifty obese patients in a study. The idea was for them to lose 10 percent of their body weight as in the experiments of Leibel and Rosenbaum, after which he would examine how hormone levels had changed. But unlike the studies of his colleagues, Proietto also measured a number of hormones produced in the gut. These included ghrelin, which stimulates appetite, and peptides YY (sometimes called PYY), GLP-1, and cholecystokinin (CCK), all of which inhibit hunger and feeding.

The participants in Proietto's study went on an extremely low-calorie diet, replacing meals with Optifast shakes and low-starch vegetables. They ate just 500–550 calories per day for eight weeks. In the ninth and tenth weeks, participants who had lost 10 percent of their body weight gradually started eating everyday foods. They were given counseling by a dietitian and a meal and exercise plan to maintain their hard-won weight loss for the next year. Proietto recommended carbohydrates with a low glycemic index such as vegetables and whole grains (the glycemic index is a way of ranking food on a scale from 1 to 100 based on its ability to affect blood-sugar levels), as well as reduced fats and thirty minutes of daily exercise. The participants would be counseled in person every two months and by phone more frequently, for a year.

Most of the subjects started at over two hundred pounds and lost an average of thirty pounds in ten weeks. The long period of consuming shakes challenged the patients, but they reveled in their weight loss and looked forward to the possibilities of being even thinner. But only a few months later, their weight started creeping back up. By the end of one year participants had regained an average of 30 to 40 percent of the weight. It was a typical effect, one recognizable to dieters everywhere.

Along the way, Proietto and his team had been taking blood samples and monitoring the participants' hormone levels in response to their changing weight. The patients' body measurements, appetite, and hormone levels were checked at the beginning, before they went on the diet, to create a baseline; then again at week 10, right after the diet; and lastly, one year after the diet.

Proietto correlated the changes in patients' weights to the measurements of their hormone levels at the various points in time. He noticed something both fascinating and sobering—his patients' hormone levels seemed to have been permanently altered in a way that actually made weight gain easier after a successful diet. The hormones were reprogramming the participants' bodies to be hungrier after they had lost weight than before, driving them to regain fat.

Leptin, the body's satiation hormone, was at its lowest level right after the initial diet ended, meaning people were feeling hungrier than they had been before starting the weight loss. And one year later, leptin levels were still significantly lower than before the diet began. Ghrelin, the hormone that makes us feel hungry, was about 20 percent higher than it had been at the outset. Peptide YY, which suppresses hunger, was much lower than before dieting. GLP-1 and cholecystokinin were also altered in a way that made people hungrier than before, and they remained that way even after the subjects had regained much of the weight they had lost.

Proietto realized the discouraging truth: combined changes in hormones were working together to make successful dieters crave food much more after they lost weight than before, inducing them to regain lost pounds. "There is a coordinated defense mechanism with multiple components all directed toward making us put on weight," Proietto said. "This is why dieters have a struggle with keeping weight off and obesity treatments fail."

Proietto's work supported Leibel's studies showing the resistant nature of fat. Our bodies will involve hormones and neural systems in order to maintain our current weight. Sustaining a lower weight is a formidable challenge.

It's in the Blood

Rudy Leibel, Michael Rosenbaum, and Joseph Proietto showed the many ways fat preserves itself. Through leptin, it can increase or decrease hormone levels, influence skeletal muscle and the nervous system, stimulate the mind to want more food, all in a concerted effort to reduce energy expenditure and sharply increase intake. But other researchers discovered another strange phenomenon. Fat, it appeared, could create a blood supply in order to promote its own growth.

The concept of angiogenesis, meaning the formation of new blood vessels, was pioneered by Harvard professor Judah Folkman, as described in chapter 3. His work showed how tumors grow and spread by sending chemical signals to nearby veins, prompting the veins to sprout new, tube-like structures, which grow in the direction of the tumor. These sprouting vessels feed and nourish the tumor with blood, allowing it to grow. The discovery led to the development of powerful drugs that block angiogenesis, prevent tumor growth, and ultimately extend the life of many cancer patients.

More recently, researchers have learned that fat tissue can do the same thing as tumors. As fat becomes enlarged from overeating, it reacts by releasing the same chemical signals that go to nearby veins, causing them to sprout in the direction of the fat. This creates additional blood supply, which delivers nutrients and oxygen that enable the fat to thrive and ultimately produce new fat cells. These newly formed blood vessels also create additional paths for circulating triglycerides to be deposited into fat tissue. Indeed, fat begets fat.

Dr. Jian-Wei Gu at the Cancer Institute at the University of Mississippi Medical Center tested the antiangiogenic drugs used to stop cancer to see if they would inhibit the blood vessel formation that enabled fat growth. Gu and his team administered an antiangiogenic drug to obese mice and they lost a whopping 70 percent of their fat mass. Their lean mass, such as muscle, stayed intact. In addition to losing fat, the animals' appetite diminished. Gu says, "This could be a very good strategy for treating obesity, at least in the short-term." Of course, efficacy and side effects of using cancer drugs in this way would have to be assessed, but Gu's research displays the massive power of one of fat's tools.

Tales of the Liposucked

Liposuction has been thought of as a surefire method to lose fat for good. If you have tried to diet and not been successful, or have a particular area of stubborn fat, you can have it liposuctioned right out of you and never worry about it again. Right? Wrong.

Recent studies show that fat can grow right back after liposuction, and not necessarily in the same place it came from. Doctors Teri Hernandez and Robert Eckel at the University of Colorado studied the effect of liposuction on thirty-two women. They separated the women into two groups—one that received liposuction in the hips, thighs, and subcutaneous fat of the lower abdomen, and a second that did not receive any treatment at all. Both groups agreed not to make any lifestyle changes for one year, during which their measurements were taken.

After six weeks, the total body fat in the liposuction group fell by about 2 percent and only nominally in the control group. But after six months, the gap diminished; after one year there was no significant difference at all between the fat of the two groups. For the women in the group who had liposuction, fat grew back to the same total percentage as before, despite the fact that they made no lifestyle changes. But fat didn't just return to the area where it had been. It moved. Some of the subcutaneous fat that had been taken from the hips, thighs, and lower abdomen resurfaced in the more dangerous visceral area, pressing close to the internal organs. In the end, the women who had liposuction ended up just as fat as before, but with less healthy fat.

Even if we try the most invasive method of fat control imaginable—surgically removing it—fat finds a way to outfox us and grow back in even more dangerous forms. What can one do to manage such a phenomenon?

Doctors Fabiana Benatti and Antonio Lancha at the University of São Paulo in Brazil examined the effects of exercise on postliposuction women. In their study, they performed liposuction on thirty-six women, removing subcutaneous fat from the lower abdomen. After liposuction, they split the women into two groups. One went back to their normal lives, the second was given a three-times-a-week workout plan consisting of a five-minute warm-up followed by thirty minutes of strength exercises and thirty to forty minutes of aerobic exercise on a treadmill. This went on for four months.

This is where the results got interesting. The abdominal subcutaneous fat (under the skin) stayed away in both groups. But the group that did not exercise gained the fat back in the visceral area (under the stomach wall) within six months, just like those in the University of Colorado study. Furthermore, this group's metabolism slowed down and they expended less energy. As Leibel and Rosenbaum had shown, once fat is gone, even by surgery, it comes back by lowering energy expenditure.

On the other hand, the group that exercised maintained their fat loss at the six-month mark and their energy expenditure remained steady. Their lean mass (meaning muscle and bone) also increased, which presumably helped maintain their energy expenditure, because lean tissue has a higher resting metabolism than fat.

The difference between the two groups was not due to food intake, since both maintained the same eating habits before liposuction as after. Apparently it was exercise alone that made the difference and maintained the fat loss. Which raises the question: if the patients had just exercised from the start, would they have needed liposuction at all?

Outfoxed by Fat?

Survival skills. Mind control. Reprogramming. Jason Bourne? No, it's your fat. Fat has an amazing ability to fight for survival. If any military in the world had such beguiling powers, it would be a force to reckon with. The same is true of fat. Anyone who has tried to get rid of extra poundage knows exactly how hard it is to do. What goes up fights to stay up, and possibly forever.

It is not impossible to fight back against fat, but it takes a great deal of effort. Ongoing lack of satisfaction is one of the most difficult situations to tolerate on a daily basis. The force of those feelings is the reason fat creeps back—we eventually give in.

There are a few ways to deal with fat's wiliness. One way is to mediate hunger and get sufficient sleep. Lack of sleep is associated with low leptin and high ghrelin levels, a combination that increases hunger, reduces satiation, and leads to obesity. Research shows that about seven hours of sleep per night balances our hormones, keeping our leptin high and ghrelin low throughout the day.

When you do eat after a good night's rest, take in plenty of water and low-calorie fiber, as provided in leafy green salads. Food volume causes the stomach to stretch, which is a signal to lower ghrelin release and decrease hunger. Also, research shows that eating soluble fiber (found in onions, garlic, leeks, bananas, barley, rye, and legumes) lowers ghrelin levels in our circulation. Add to that salad some protein and fats, which are known to release CCK and PYY, the two hormones released from the gut that enhance satiation. Adding strength-building exercises can offset the muscle efficiency and slowing of metabolism that occurs after losing fat because additional muscle will burn more calories.

The main tool to ensure long-term weight loss is persistence. Once you've gained weight and need to lose it, your challenge is harder than that of someone who's only maintaining a weight they are at naturally. Just as fat is wily, clever, and tenacious, you will need the same qualities to fight it back. Given the right motivations, long-term weight loss can be accomplished (more on this in chapter 10). After all, even Jason Bourne takes it on the chin sometimes.

II

IT IS NOT ONLY FOOD
THAT MAKES US
FAT

Chapter 6

Bacteria and Viruses— Microscopic in Size, Giant in Effect

Randy is sixty-two years old and stands tall at six foot one. He grew up on a farm in Glasford, Illinois, in the 1950s. Glasford is a peaceful, quiet place, with intensely hot summers, beautiful crisp autumns, and the stinging cold winters typical of the Midwest. Randy was raised with the strong discipline of a farming family. From the time he was five, he would get out of bed at dawn, and before breakfast he'd put on his boots and jeans to milk cows, lift hay, and clean the chicken coops. Day in and out, no matter the weather or how he felt, Randy did his physically demanding chores. Only when his work was complete would he come into the kitchen for breakfast.

Tending to the chickens was hard work—it involved getting into the pen, clearing birds out of their dirty cages, and shooing them into a holding enclosure. This process was always a little scary because the animals could be quite aggressive after being cooped up all night. On one of these occasions, when Randy was eleven, a particularly large and perturbed rooster swung its claw and gave him a good spurring on his leg. Randy felt the piercing of his skin and squealed in pain. He said it felt like being gored by a thick fishhook. The rooster left a long gash, and blood streamed down Randy's leg to his ankle. He ran back to the house to clean the wound, as chickens are filthy after a night in their cages.

Some days later, Randy noticed a change in his appetite. He was constantly hungry. He felt drawn to food and thought about it all the time. He started eating in between meals and overeating when he finally sat down to dinner. Randy had always been a skinny kid, but in the course of the next year, he gained about ten pounds. His parents thought it might be puberty, though it seemed a little early. His pudginess was also unusual given that everyone else in the family was thin. Randy was no stranger to discipline. He forced himself to eat less, switched to lower-calorie foods and exercised more. But by the time he was a teenager, he was bouncing between thirty and forty pounds overweight. He says, "I gained all of this weight even though these were some of my most active years on the farm."

Randy successfully lost weight for special occasions, such as an important student council meeting or the prom, but he was terrified to take his shirt off for swimming or gym class. He says, "The only goal I had that took most of my brain power after age fourteen was to lose weight. I did everything possible to not eat. That was the life I lived." He lamented that while he was strong enough to do any physical task, his body would never take on a classic male V-shaped physique.

Randy's family supported his efforts to control his weight. They made lower-calorie foods, gave him time to exercise, and didn't pressure him to eat things he didn't want. However, he continued to struggle with his weight through college. He says, "I was up and down between 200 and 230 pounds or so in my early twenties, and it was a huge fight." Randy kept thinking back to the moment everything changed. He had been the skinniest kid among his friends. And then he got cut by that chicken.

The Curious Case of Indian Chickens

In Mumbai, India, Nikhil Dhurandhar followed his father Vinod's footsteps in treating obesity. For the elder Dr. Dhurandhar, treating the obese had been a life's commitment. Vinod himself had been overweight at one time, but through restricting food, planning his meals, and taking up tennis he lost sixty pounds, to get down to 140. He figured that if he could accomplish this for himself, he could help others. He started a medical practice specializing in the treatment of obesity and it quickly grew. Nikhil was inspired by his father and aimed to join his practice some-day. Nikhil recounts, "In conversations around the dinner table growing up, I heard a lot about obesity, how obese individuals are taken for a ride by quacks, and how much they suffer. That got me interested in the field." The younger Dhurandhar went to medical school and then joined his father before branching out on his own. Eventually, he started three clinics and treated over ten thousand patients.

But Nikhil ran into the same obstacle that had bedeviled obesity doctors everywhere. "The problem was that I was not able to pro-duce something for patients that could have meaningful weight loss that was sustainable for a long time," he says. "Patients kept coming back. . . . It is as Albert Stunkard of the University of Pennsylvania once said, 'Most obese persons will not stay in treatment, most will not lose weight, and of those who do lose weight, most will regain it.' Sadly, that was true."

Many doctors might have accepted the maxim, but not Nikhil Dhurandhar. An inquisitive and thoughtful person who needs answers, he explains that his enduring combination of curiosity and ignorance (or lack of awareness of ingrained scientific beliefs) enable him to ask questions when others don't.

These opposing traits first emerged when he was a child. In third grade, Dhurandhar watched a cordon of ants carrying food crumbs larger than their bodies. He questioned why the ants didn't just eat the crumbs instead of carrying them. The tiny insects crawled from one end of the room to another, struggling to carry their cargo, but not even one stopped to eat it. Did ants eat at all, or did they just carry food from one place to another? he wondered. The young Dhurandhar designed his first experiment: he took a handful of ants, put them in a box with some rice, then buried them, planning to dig them up after a few days to see if any of the rice was ingested. Unfortunately, the ants died, but Dhurandhar's curiosity, particu-larly regarding food, stayed alive.

Now as a doctor addressing obesity, Dhurandhar was driven to ask probing questions about obesity and the way it was treated. He decided to go to the United States to do graduate work and get training in nutrition. He says, "If I wanted to spend my career in obesity, I needed to be better equipped. So I took off from my practice, came to the United States, finished my master's here in eleven months, in a hurry, and went back to Mumbai to join a PhD program in biochemistry. I continued with my patients, however, treating them and pursuing research at the same time."

Dhurandhar explains how his life would take fateful turns from this point forward, as if someone was guiding him as he sought answers to obesity. Particularly notable was the number three. This is how many times that fate intervened to change his life, and the number of trusted scientific principles he would break in his career.

The first time fate intervened in Dhurandhar's life was when he was meeting his father and a family friend, S. M. Ajinkya, a veterinary pathologist, for tea. Ajinkya described an epidemic then blazing through the Indian poultry industry killing thousands of chickens. He had identified the virus and named it using, in part, his own initials—SMAM-1. Upon necropsy, Ajinkya explained, the chickens were found to have shrunken thymuses, enlarged kidneys and livers, and fat deposited in the abdomen. Dhurandhar thought this was unusual because typically viruses cause weight loss, not gain. Ajinkya was about to go on, but Dhurandhar stopped him: "You just said something that doesn't sound right to me. You said that the chickens had a lot of fat in their abdomen. Is it possible that the virus was making them fat?"

Ajinkya could have dismissed Dhurandhar's curiosity, and the entire field of "infectobesity" that was inspired by this question, by simply saying, "No, that is not possible, viruses don't make people fat." It would have been the expected answer, as scientists are naturally skeptical, and there was no evidence for such a thing. But being open-minded, Ajinkya answered honestly, "I don't know," and urged Dhurandhar to study the question. That fateful conversation set Dhurandhar on a path to investigate as part of his PhD project whether a virus *could* cause fat.

He got to work immediately, setting up experiments to investigate whether the SMAM-1 virus could make chickens fat. But when he told colleagues of his plan, he faced overwhelming skepticism. Dhurandhar remembers, "People would ask, 'Why are you doing this? Nobody else has shown that viruses lead to fat.' That used to make me really mad. I said, 'Isn't that the very reason you should do the experiment?'"

Dhurandhar pushed ahead and arranged an experiment using twenty healthy chickens. He infected half of them with SMAM-1 and left the other half uninfected. During the experiment, both groups of chickens consumed the same amount of food. By the end of the experiment, only the chickens infected with the SMAM-1 virus had become fat. However, even though the infected chickens were fatter, they had lower cholesterol and triglyceride levels in their blood than the uninfected birds. "It was quite paradoxical," Dhurandhar remembers, "because if you have a fatter chicken, you would expect them to have greater cholesterol and circulating triglycerides, but instead those levels went in the wrong direction. So we have chickens that are infected with the virus that are fatter with lower cholesterol and lower triglycerides."

To confirm the results, he set up a repeat experiment, this time using one hundred chickens. Again, only the chickens with the SMAM-1 virus in their blood became fat. Dhurandhar was intrigued. A virus, it seemed, was causing obesity. If that was the case, could fat be contagious? Dhurandhar thought of a way to test this. He arranged three groups of chickens in separate cages: one group that was not infected, a second group that was infected with the virus, and a third group that caged infected and uninfected chickens together. Within three weeks, the uninfected chickens that shared a cage with infected ones had caught the virus and gained a significant amount of body fat compared to the isolated uninfected birds. Dhurandhar says, "We didn't infect these chickens. It was a horizontal infection within the same species, and they gained more than double the amount of fat, but their cholesterol and triglycerides dropped." Fat, it seemed, could indeed be contagious.

Now, Dhurandhar is a man of science. He is rational and calm. But even he had to admit that the idea that fat can be infectious was startling. Does this mean that sneezing on somebody can transmit obesity? This now seemed possible in animals, but what about humans? Injecting the virus into people would be unethical, but Dhurandhar did have a way to test patients to see if they had contracted the virus in the past.

Dhurandhar says, "At that time I had my obesity clinic, and I was doing blood tests for patients for their treatment. I thought I might just as well take a little bit of blood and test for antibodies to SMAM-1. Antibodies would indicate whether the patient was infected in the past with SMAM-1. The conventional wisdom is that an adenovirus* for chickens does not infect humans, but I decided to check anyway. It turned out that 20 percent of the people we tested were positive for antibodies for SMAM-1. And those 20 percent were heavier, had greater body mass index and lower cholesterol and lower triglycerides compared to the antibody-negative individuals, just as the chickens had." Dhurandhar observed that people who had been infected with SMAM-1 were on average thirty-three pounds heavier than those who weren't infected.

In addition to this thirty-three, the number three was making an appearance in other ways. Dhurandhar's findings violated three tenets of conventional wisdom in science: (1) that viruses cannot cause weight gain; (2) that higher levels of fat cause an increase in circulating cholesterol and triglycerides; and (3) that a chicken adenovirus cannot infect humans. He says, "At that point we had violated conventional wisdom so many times that I have very little regard for conventional wisdom anymore."

The Pounds Keep Coming

While Nikhil Dhurandhar was in India pursuing his curiosity about fat, Randy was looking for solutions of his own. After a brief stint as a teacher he moved back to the family land in 1977 because he loved farming. As he approached his thirties, he was pushing 280 pounds. "I worked harder physically than I ever had at any time in my life after I moved to the farm, and that was the part of my weight cycle where the gains were in the upper quadrant of the 270 to 300

*Viruses originally discovered in adenoid tissue, a mass of soft tissue that sits behind the nasal cavity; SMAM-1 is categorized as one.

and back and forth," he says. "If I got to 250 for a brief few days I might look thin, but 280 was just a few weeks away. I should have been able to have a teaspoon of dessert and not have it destroy me. But the fact of the matter is that I couldn't. The smallest indulgence would make me put on the pounds immediately."

In those years Randy married and had four children. At family dinners and holiday gatherings, he ate alongside everyone else, but tried eating less than the others. Still, his weight ballooned; by his late thirties he had topped 300 pounds. He remembers feeling hungry all the time, though even when he abstained it didn't help him lose weight. "I could have several good weeks of eating stringently, much less than others around me, but if I went off my diet for just one meal—boom, the weight would come back."

Randy clearly had a biological propensity for accumulating fat, but he also felt that his environment was a problem. "People just want you to be like them," he says. "They want you to eat like them, do like them. I tried to partake, but I knew my body just gained fat easier than others. When you don't want to eat with them, people think you don't like them. Not only that, but I felt hungrier than others most of the time. For me to be around food and have to eat like others did was like a bullet in my body. I couldn't eat the way other people did and stay thin. My body is just different." The effort to control his eating, even when it was successful, made Randy miserable: "I can't tell you what it is like to be hungry all the time. It is an ongoing stress. Try it. Most people who give advice don't have to feel it."

Coming to America

Dhurandhar felt confident about his findings that the SMAM-1 virus could cause fat in humans, so he submitted his research for publication in the scientific literature. Many journals rejected the work simply because the editors didn't believe it. A virus causing fat was just too farfetched. Moreover, Dhurandhar didn't know the exact mechanism of how the virus caused the obesity, only that there was a correlation. Ingrained belief that viruses were unrelated to fat caused many to simply deny the raw data. Some of Dhurandhar's studies underwent years of rejection before any journal would agree to publish them.

Dhurandhar received his PhD from the University of Bombay in 1992 and resumed treating obesity patients in India. However, his thinking had changed permanently. The treatment of obesity held less interest for him now and he had a new passion to investigate the connection between viruses and obesity. He'd heard of an online database called Medline, which allowed scientists to search their colleagues' publications. (Medline, now called PubMed, is the essential source for online literature research, used by every scientist.) However, in the early 1990s, Internet connections were not widely available in India, so Dhurandhar wrote a letter to the National Library of Medicine in the United States asking them to conduct a search for relevant papers. Today, such a search would take minutes at most. At the time, he had to wait several weeks for the results.

Dhurandhar found out that others had also been researching the topic. One publication on canine distemper virus that causes obesity in mice was reported in *Science* in 1982. A second paper focused on Rous-associated virus (RAV), which also causes obesity in chickens. Dhurandhar was both relieved and worried. Had someone already scooped his research? "It was a good thing and a bad thing," he says. "It is a bad thing in that somebody had already discovered that a virus can cause obesity, but a good thing in that I was not the only fool. I was the only one working on adenoviruses, however, and that made me ecstatic."

Even better, no one had yet studied whether viruses could cause obesity in humans. It was a gripping question and Dhurandhar couldn't get it out of his head. The curiosity overtook every spare moment. He finally decided to relinquish his successful medical practice to devote himself to the topic. And he knew that if he were serious about pursuing the research, he would need to leave India for the United States.

Dhurandhar started writing to people there and making phone calls in search of a postdoctoral position, but, he says, "I couldn't understand the response that I got from the U.S. The bottom line was they said to 'go away,' to put it politely. I guess I can understand it in hindsight. Not only is some unknown guy from a weird country writing to you about a completely weird topic that a virus causes obesity, but he wants to come to your lab, and use your money to advance his research. Usually when people come to a lab as postdoctoral fellow, they don't bring in their own projects, they work on projects that are assigned to them. But I wanted to do it the other way."

Dhurandhar was having no luck getting to the U.S. on a postdoc. But his passion remained. He decided to try another angle. He says, "I decided I'm going to move to the U.S. and take any postdoctoral position that comes my way. When I'm in the U.S., I'll be at least on the same planet. And then I'll try to contact people and convince them from there."

So Dhurandhar and his wife, with their seven-year-old son, took a leap of faith. They put their lives into three suitcases and came to the U.S. Dhurandhar ended up in a postdoc in North Dakota cutting sunflowers for a project to study pectin. He says, "We gave ourselves two years to find a postdoctorate position to work with viruses and obesity. If it didn't happen, we would go back to India and I would resume my practice."

Once in the U.S., Dhurandhar contacted every lab that might be interested in his work. He made phone calls, tried introductions through friends, and wrote letters—thirty or forty at a time—and gave them to his wife to mail. But in two years, no one was interested. Exhausted and dispirited, Dhurandhar and his wife decided to return to India. They enrolled their son at an Indian school and made preparations to go back. Dhurandhar says, "I did not wish to continue living in the U.S. if I could not work on viruses and obesity."

But fate intervened a second time in Dhurandhar's career. Richard Atkinson at the University of Wisconsin Medical School was an established obesity scientist. He had read the paper Dhurandhar published while still living in India. Atkinson developed an interest in virology and obesity when he learned, in 1982, that canine distemper virus (CDV) caused fat in mice (one of the same papers Dhurandhar received from the National Library of Medicine). He wanted to know whether measles, which is similar in structure to CDV, was having the same effect on children. However, when he requested a grant from the Centers for Disease Control to study it, he was denied.

Atkinson was disappointed, but no less intrigued. He kept a watchful eye on the subject. Then one day Dhurandhar contacted him out of the blue. Atkinson was a well-known researcher and previous head of the North American Association for the Study of Obesity (now called The Obesity Society), so he was used to getting calls from eager postdocs looking for work. However, Atkinson says, "Usually the research of PhD students is assigned to them by their principal investigator, but as I spoke to Nikhil it became apparent that despite the numerous authors on his publications, he had been driving his own research on obesity all throughout his PhD." Atkinson was also deeply impressed by Dhurandhar's sacrifice. Atkinson recalls, "Dhurandhar had three obesity clinics in India, he had a thriving medical practice. Yet he gave it all up. He took a 95 percent pay cut to come to the U.S. as a postdoc and pursue research in obesity. He is a true scientist."

Only weeks before Dhurandhar was planning to move back to India, Atkinson offered him a job at the University of Wisconsin, Madison. In 1994, Dhurandhar moved there as a postdoctoral fellow.

A Weight Plan for Diabetics

In the fall of 1989, Randy applied for a commercial driver's license. The application required a medical exam. After his urine test, the nurse asked Randy if he felt all right. "Normal for the day," he replied. But the nurse told Randy he would have to give a blood sample because she thought the lab had spilled glucose solution into his urine sample. The blood work showed that Randy's glucose level was near 500 mg/dL (recall that a normal reading is 100). The lab hadn't made a mistake with the urine sample after all; Randy's numbers were just off the charts. Alarmed, the nurse notified Randy's doctor, who then tested him for fasting blood sugar levels. The results showed that Randy had insulin resistance and severe diabetes.

At forty years old and 350 pounds, Randy was in trouble. He was constantly hungry and continuing to gain weight. If he didn't fix this problem soon, he would start to develop serious complications of diabetes, including cardiovascular disease and nerve damage.

Having tried and failed multiple diets, Randy and his doctor decided the best hope was a hospital program for severe diabetics. The staff tested Randy's blood frequently to determine the optimal dosage and timing of insulin injections to regulate his blood sugar. Randy learned about the Diabetic Exchange diet, which allots patients a specific number of servings of meat, carbohydrates, vegetables, and fat. He cut out all refined carbohydrates, including bread. He says, "I haven't had a slice of bread or piece of pizza in years."

But would even this program be enough? Randy had always had a difficult time controlling his weight, though not for lack of trying. He had been fighting fat since his childhood by controlling portions, exercising, and avoiding social eating. But his discipline was no match for his own fat. Randy had to get his weight under control permanently. The hospital environment was helpful. Randy started losing weight. However, despite strictly adhering to the diet, he only dropped a few pounds.

The Virus in Americans

After being a postdoctoral fellow at Madison, Dhurandhar was excited to finally be at liberty to pursue what he loved. He had an intense curiosity about viruses and was eager to get started finding answers. However, when he tried to get samples of the SMAM-1 virus that he had worked with in India, the U.S. Department of Agriculture refused to grant him an import license. It had taken Dhurandhar two years to finally get a postdoc and now he couldn't get the virus he needed. He was deeply disappointed, but fate would intervene a third time.

Unable to get SMAM-1, Dhurandhar approached a company that sells viruses for research. Their catalog listed some fifty human adenoviruses. He says, "I was going to order *the* human adenovirus, but there was no *the* adenovirus—there were fifty different human adenoviruses! So I was stuck again. I wondered how do I go about this? Should we start number one, number two, number three, number fifty, forty-nine, forty-eight? So [with] a little bit of guesswork and mostly luck, we decided to work with number thirty-six. We liked number thirty-six because it was antigenically unique—meaning it did not cross react with other viruses in the group, and antibodies to other viruses would not neutralize it."

That was a serendipitous choice. It turned out that Ad-36 had similar qualities to SMAM-1 in chickens. Atkinson thought Ad-36 might very well be a mutated form of SMAM-1. When Dhurandhar infected chickens with Ad-36, their fat increased and their cholesterol and triglycerides decreased, just as had happened with SMAM-1. Dhurandhar wanted to make sure he was not getting a false positive, so he injected another group of chickens with a virus called CELO to ensure that other viruses were not also producing fat in chickens. Additionally, he maintained a group of chickens who had not been injected with anything. When he compared the three groups—one group infected with Ad-36, one infected with CELO, and one group not infected—only the Ad-36 group became fatter. Dhurandhar then tried the experiments in mice and marmosets. In every case, Ad-36 made animals fatter. Marmosets gained about three times as much weight as the uninfected animals, their body fat increasing by almost 60 percent!

Now came the big question: would Ad-36 have any effect on humans? Dhurandhar and Atkinson tested over five hundred human subjects to see if they had antibodies to the Ad-36 virus, indicating they had been infected with it at some point in their lives. His team found that 30 percent of subjects who were obese tested positive for Ad-36, but only 11 percent of nonobese individuals did—a 3 to 1 ratio. In addition, nonobese individuals who tested positive for Ad-36 were significantly heavier than those who had never been exposed to the virus. Once again, the virus was correlated with fat.

Next, Dhurandhar devised an even more stringent experiment. He tested pairs of twins for presence of Ad-36. He explains, "Our hypothesis was that twins have similar weights. But if we focus on twin pairs, one of whom is positive for virus antibodies and one who is negative, we have a discordant twin pair. And if the virus has anything to do with human obesity, the antibody-positive co-twin will be heavier than its antibody-negative counterpart co-twin. So we tested the blood, and before we knew it we had 28 sets of twins there who were discordant for viral infection, so 56 people. And it turned out exactly the way we hypothesized—the Ad-36 positive co-twins were significantly fatter compared to their Ad-36 negative counterparts."

Of course, it's unethical to infect human subjects with viruses for research, so the study can't be perfectly confirmed. But, Dhurandhar says, "This is the closest you can come to showing the role of the virus in humans, short of infecting them."

A New Way to Manage Fat—Stop the Blame

Randy's physician had been treating him for years and knew that his patient's struggle was difficult and ongoing. Since his hospital stay, Randy had done better at controlling his weight, but he needed more specialized treatment to succeed long term. The physician referred Randy to an endocrinologist—Richard Atkinson at the University of Wisconsin, in Madison—who was having some success with difficult obesity cases.

Randy went to see Dr. Atkinson, knowing that if he didn't get his fat under control, it was going to kill him. The first thing Randy noticed about Atkinson was that he was kind. He didn't make Randy feel guilty about his weight. "Other places put the blame on you," Randy says. "They go back into your past, what did you do to get here. It is very judgmental. Atkinson did none of that. He said okay we are here now, how do we fix it? He was very future oriented."

Atkinson had designed a long-term program to treat obesity. He explained to his patients that obesity is a chronic disease and they would be in treatment "forever." In the first three months of the program, patients would meet several days per week and attend a lecture explaining obesity and the underpinnings of fat. After that, visits decreased to one every one to two weeks, then one every one to two months. Those who started regaining weight were asked to resume more frequent visits. Subjects had to commit to the full program in order to enroll. The idea of finally learning the science of fat excited Randy. He says, "As soon as I heard about university lectures and learning about my condition, I said, 'Sign me up!' I would drive all the way from Illinois to Madison, Wisconsin, just for this class, and it was worth it."

In the lectures, Atkinson explained the scientific research into obesity—what was known with certainty and what was not. He explained set point theory—the body's efforts to maintain a constant weight, and the extreme effort that is required to change it. He described landmark experiments in which lean subjects who gained an average of 25 percent body mass had to eat abundantly more to maintain it than those who were obese. He explained the research on Ad-36, and how a virus can be correlated with fatness. The scientific perspective helped Randy understand fat's many defense mechanisms, and the strategies he would need to conquer it.

Atkinson also introduced Randy to his new postdoctoral assistant, a young scientist from India, Dr. Nikhil Dhurandhar. Dhurandhar examined Randy and studied his blood samples. Randy tested positive for antibodies to Ad-36, meaning he had likely been infected with the virus at some point in the past. Randy remembered being scratched by that rooster as a child, and that afterward his appetite exploded and he started gaining weight quickly. His troubles with food and rapid fat accumulation—he understood it all now. If he was like the chickens, the marmosets, the twins, and the other humans in the study, then his infection with Ad-36 was helping his body to accumulate fat. He says, "What Atkinson and Dhurandhar did for me changed my life. They made everything make sense. It was very liberating and very empowering."

How Does a Virus Lead To Fat?

How would a virus like Ad-36 cause fat? Atkinson explains, "There are three ways that we think Ad-36 makes people fatter: (1) It increases the uptake of glucose from the blood and converts it to fat; (2) it increases the creation of fat molecules through fatty acid synthase, an enzyme that creates fat; and (3) it enables the creation of more fat cells to hold all the fat by committing stem cells, which can turn into either bone or fat, into fat. So the fat cells that exist are getting bigger, and the body is creating more of them."

The researchers acknowledge that the rooster scratch may have been the start of Randy's infection. But they are cautious—the transmissibility of Ad-36 from chickens to humans has never directly been studied.

Although Dhurandhar has left the University of Wisconsin to head the Nutritional Sciences department at Texas Tech University, and Atkinson has moved to Virginia, the two stay closely in touch. Recently, Dhurandhar has followed 1,500 subjects over a ten-year period, testing them for antibodies for Ad-36 at the beginning of the study, and checking yearly. He says, "It turns out that antibody-positive people who were positive at the beginning gained significantly greater body mass over ten years." Atkinson did a similar study, assessing the blood serum at the time of entry of U.S. Air Force personnel from 1995 until 2012. Those who were nonobese at the time of entry into the service and were also infected with the Ad-36 virus had an almost fourfold higher risk of being overweight by the end of the study.

Though Dhurandhar and Atkinson have conducted several strong studies showing the contribution of Ad-36 to fatness, skepticism remains. Atkinson says, "I remember giving a talk at a conference where I presented fifteen different studies in which Ad-36 either caused or was correlated to fatness. At the end of it, a good friend said to me, 'I just don't believe it.' He didn't give a reason; he just didn't believe it. People are really stuck on eating and exercise as the only contributors to fatness. But there is more to it."

Dhurandhar has had similar experiences and adds, "There's a difference between science and faith. What you believe belongs in faith and not in science. In science you have to go by data. I have faced people who are skeptical, but when I ask them why, they can't pinpoint a specific reason. Science is not about belief, it is about fact. There is a saying—'In God we trust, all others bring data.'"

Sometimes Science Is Hard to Swallow

Skepticism about paradigm-shifting ideas is common in science. Barry Marshall was another researcher who faced disbelief regarding his hypothesis that the bacteria *Helicobacter pylori*, and not stress, was the cause of ulcers. Pharmaceutical companies were making billions from the belief that emotional turmoil prompted the release of excessive stomach acids that could only be relieved with blockbuster drugs such as Tagamet and Zantac. But the ulcers would come back as soon as patients stopped taking antacids—regardless of stress. Worse, the ulcers sometimes progressed to stomach cancer.

Marshall's colleague Robin Warren, a pathologist at the Royal Perth Hospital, saw in his own microscope that ulcers were accompanied by an abundance of the corkscrew-shaped *H. pylori* bacteria. Marshall became an evangelist, trying to get the word out to physicians. But he was met with incredulity by the scientific community, and ultimately was refused funding to study the bacteria further. Unable to secure a patient for a clinical trial, he finally tested the only subject who was willing to participate—himself. He drank a cocktail of *H. pylori* to prove his point, and shortly afterward started vomiting and developed the early stages of ulcers. He had researched antibiotics capable of killing the bacteria. So he quickly took the drugs and cured his ulcers.

Even when Marshall publicized his story, he didn't get much traction in his native Australia. But in the U.S. press, which has an affection for eye-catching headlines, his tale started to catch on. The attention was not necessarily the type a scientist craves—headlines like "Guinea-Pig Doctor Experiments on Self and Cures Ulcer" ran in tabloids such as the *National Enquirer*, but the publicity got the attention of the U.S. Food and Drug Administration, which urged a full clinical trial on the treatment of ulcers with antibiotics. The trial was successful and Marshall and Warren were finally proven right. They won the Nobel Prize in 2005 for their discovery, a sweet vindication after years of professional ostracism.

Dhurandhar hopes new research will overcome skepticism about infectobesity as it did for *H. pylori*. Perhaps as scientists gain more insight on the inner workings of the virus and are able to further pinpoint its molecular mechanism, this skepticism will abate. Currently, the idea of fat being enabled by bacteria and viruses flies in the face of centuries of common wisdom that obesity stems only from overeating and sloth. Disbelief remains strong even though canine distemper virus, Rous-associated virus type 7 (RAV-7), and Borna virus all cause fatness in animals. Dhurandhar says, "There have been eighteen to twenty studies done by various labs that have shown a significant association of Ad-36 with obesity in humans, no matter what race."

Richard Atkinson anticipates the development of a vaccine against Ad-36. He thinks that 30 percent of obese people are affected by this virus and are heavier because of it. He would like to see a day when children get vaccinated for Ad-36 as they do now for chickenpox and measles. But for the moment there is no direct treatment for Ad-36. Atkinson says, "Even if you have had the virus, and are predisposed for fatness, what you eat and how much you exercise is still in your control. You may just have to work harder at it."

Randy certainly works harder than most. He managed to get his weight down from 350 pounds to 170. But it wasn't easy. He limits his intake to 1,200–1,500 calories per day, about half of what an adult male normally eats. His major meal is a green salad, and he has some fruit and nut snacks through the day. Atkinson says of Randy, "He is a remarkable person, with more discipline than anyone I have ever met."

Randy divides people into the "eating world" and the "noneating world." He says, "I just can't eat what others eat. I have to tell my family and friends, if you want me to be alive, don't expect me to eat with you. My family has been very supportive and that is key. If we go out, everyone will eat what they want, but I'll stick to my fruit and nuts, or bring boiled eggs with me. You have to realize you are not part of the 'eating world.'"

Randy is happier now than he has been in years. He has learned about his condition and fights every day to keep his weight in check. He has even mortgaged his house to pay for gastric bypass surgery, just to make sure his weight doesn't come back. Insurance wouldn't pay because at 225 pounds he wasn't heavy enough. He says, "Some people gain weight just so they can get the surgery, then they've ruined their eating habits to where even after the surgery, they now can't keep off the weight. If you don't have good eating habits coming in, the surgery won't be durable. . . . I look better now than I have in a long time. In fact, friends who were thinner than me earlier in life are now heavier than me." Randy's goal used to be to be able to suck in his gut enough so his fat didn't show. Now, he says, "I'm a clap-along jogger of sixty-two who for the first time in his life might have the courage to take his shirt off in gym class. . . . My goal now is to get to 160 pounds and then get into a Speedo!"

It's Not Just Viruses; Bacteria
Can Cause Fat Too

Randy's relationship with food is unusual, but he is hardly unique in feeling that he eats next to nothing and still gains weight. Many people feel this way—their peers eat a three-course meal, they only eat half a course, and yet they end up fatter. Their peers may not be taller or more muscular, some don't even exercise, yet they just don't get fat. For the weight-challenged, it's like being possessed by a fat-loving alien, and this may not be far from the truth. But it is not just one alien: it is trillions of them. Today, medical science is paying close attention to the microbes we all contain, such as the bacteria and viruses we pick up along the way that affect our physical well-being in numerous ways, including how much fat we store.

It's an uncomfortable thought: when it comes to fat, we are not alone.

Antonie van Leeuwenhoek was one of the first observers of body microbes. In 1683, he scraped plaque off his teeth and examined the substance under his microscope, observing hundreds of small "animalcules" darting around on his lens. It seemed odd to him that when he drank hot coffee, they would die.

In recent decades our knowledge of bacteria has increased tremendously. We now know that these single-cell organisms are everywhere. From the time we are born, they start to colonize our nasal path, armpits, skin, lungs, mouth, digestive tract—almost any body part that has exposure to the outside world. They cohabit with us, residing in our bodies in a symbiotic fashion, helping themselves and often helping us.

Just going through the birth canal, which is rife with microbes, coats a newborn with bacteria. Even in a Caesarean delivery, the bacteria on the mother's skin will attach to the new baby. The method of early feeding—breast versus bottle—also affects the type of early bacteria we take on. Either way, the bacteria of a child tends to correlate with those of a parent, especially in the gut. The increased exposure to the environment in our first few years of life increases the types and numbers of bacteria we have, and as we grow our guts come to possess around 100 trillion microbes. Ultimately, humans have ten times more one-celled microbes in our bodies than our own body cells, meaning we are actually more microbial than human.

The largest population of bacteria in our bodies lives in the lower half of our intestines and helps with energy metabolism, vitamin synthesis, and digestion. Is it any surprise that bacteria would affect our fat and weight? Depending on the type and amount of bacteria we have, we may be absorbing more or fewer calories from our food than those around us, which corresponds to more or less body weight.

Dr. Jeffrey Gordon at Washington University in St. Louis, Missouri, is one of the best-known researchers of gut bacteria. Tall, with curly brown hair and wire frame glasses, he speaks intensely in run-on sentences when describing his research. Gordon was studying the role of bacteria in metabolism when he noticed an odd trend. Working with Fredrik Bäckhed, his team raised two groups of mice: one under sterile conditions, without any bacterial growth in their bodies, the other conventionally in the open air so they harbored the typical distribution of bacteria in their intestines. The amount and type of food both groups were given was identical. The researchers then used X-ray absorptiometry* to accurately assess the amount of fat the mice had at eight to ten weeks old. The results were star-

---

*X-ray absorptiometry is a way to measure the density or mass of a material by comparing the absorption of X-rays.

tling. The mice that were raised conventionally, with the full spectrum of bacteria in their gut, had 42 percent more fat than the mice with no bacteria, even though they consumed almost a third less of their food allotment than the sterile mice. Something about the bacteria in the mice was increasing fat storage.

Gordon and his team at first thought that the sterile mice might have higher metabolic rates. But they found, to their surprise, that the bacteria-free mice had a metabolic rate that was 27 percent *lower* than that of the normal mice. The mice with the full spectrum of bacteria in their gut ate less, had higher metabolic rates, yet were significantly fatter than those without bacteria.

What would happen, Gordon wondered, if bacteria from the normal mice were transferred to the bacteria-free ones? They transferred microbes from the intestines of the conventionally raised mice into the gut of the bacteria-free mice. In fourteen days, the previously bacteria-free mice had a 57 percent increase in body fat! Even stranger, these newly infected mice were eating 27 percent *less* than the bacteria-free mice. So, once again, mice with gut bacteria were eating over a quarter less, yet were more than 50 percent fatter, than their sterile counterparts.

The effect wasn't limited to mice. A few years later, another member of Gordon's team, Vanessa Ridaura, devised a test to see if bacteria could cause weight gain in humans. The team identified four sets of twins in which one was obese and the other was lean. Gordon transplanted bacteria from the feces of each twin into a lean, bacteria-free mouse. Each recipient mouse was individually caged after transplantation so that they weren't able to transmit the newly implanted bacteria to one another. All mice were fed the same amount and type of food during the test.

Astonishingly, each mouse took on characteristics of its human fecal donor. The mouse that received bacteria from an obese twin gained significantly more fat than the mouse receiving microbes from the lean sibling. And the amount of feces produced by the mice that received bacteria from the lean twins was higher than that of the mice that got bacteria from the obese ones, indicating that the lean animals were eliminating more food as waste, even though both sets of mice were eating the same amount.

Apparently, the bacteria in lean subjects was harvesting less energy from food and eliminating more of it as waste than the bacteria in the heavy subjects. Gordon says, "We have proof from the animal studies that there might be a causal relationship because we've transplanted microbial communities from humans with obesity. And we've shown that they can transmit an increased adiposity phenotype [appearance] as well as metabolic disorders, especially in obesity."

How do bacteria extract energy and cause fat to be stored? Gut microbes have enzymes that humans don't carry. They can thus digest parts of plants that our own digestive system cannot. These enzymes allow the bacteria to break down polysaccharides (complex sugars and starches that our bodies would find nondigestible) and turn them into simple sugars that we can easily absorb. In this way, bacteria enable us to extract more calories from food than we can do on our own. In addition, bacteria increase the number of capillaries in the small intestine, which allows the increased absorption of food from the gut. So in effect bacteria change our digestion in two ways—first by improving the ability of the gut to absorb food, and then by increasing the amount of sugars extracted from food.

Bacteria's influence goes beyond digestion. Bacteria are also linked to a decrease in a protein called FIAF (Fasting-Induced Adipose Factor), which suppresses the storage of fat. By decreasing FIAF, bacteria enable fat levels to increase. All these factors combined—greater gut absorption, higher calorie extraction from food, lower levels of FIAF—explain why mice with normal bacterial distribution had more fat than those with no bacteria at all.

It is important to note that not all bacteria are the same. Some are associated with obesity, while others are not. This is a changing area of research, and new discoveries are shedding light on the complexities of our microbiome (the collective term used for all of our inhabitant microorganisms). Some studies have shown that obese individuals have a higher amount of gut bacteria called Firmicutes and a lower amount of Bacteroidetes, while lean individuals have the reverse. Certain species of Firmicutes are thought to be more efficient at breaking down starches, thus extracting more energy from food and passing less of it as waste. From an evolutionary standpoint, the potential upside is a lot less calories going out the door as waste. But nowadays, the potential downside is a lot less calories going out the door as waste! Other recent studies have shown that the diversity of bacteria in our gut is also associated with fatness, with those who are lean having a higher diversity than those who are obese. Either way, evidence is growing that our microbiome and our fat are not independent.

Jeffrey Gordon uses a bowl of cereal as a way to explain the variability in our digestive processes. Cereal is high in polysaccharides. The amount of calories we will get from that bowl depends on our bacterial profile. Some bacteria are more efficient at converting food to calories than others. So, even though the nutritional information on the package may indicate 110 calories per serving, in reality, depending on your microbes, you may get more or fewer calories. Gordon says, "The question is whether the nutritional value of a bowl of Cheerios is the same for everyone. We think it does vary, and actually to measure that carefully in human trials is something that still needs to be done."

The good news is that our bacterial distribution is not static. Studies show that when obese individuals lose weight, by restricting either carbohydrates or fats, their bacterial distribution shifts to a reduced number of Firmicutes and larger proportion of Bacteroidetes. They also increase their bacterial diversity. In this way, once again, fat begets fat—an energy-rich diet is associated with bacteria that enable even higher energy extraction from foods. But on the flip side, fat loss begets more fat loss—lower-energy foods induce weight loss and promote it further by shifting the bacteria population, causing lower energy extraction of food and more waste. Indeed, what we eat causes our weight to spiral up or down for more reasons than we might think.

Working with Your Microbiome

Microbiome research is a developing field, so most research and interpretation should be seen as preliminary. However, if you are curious to know what is in your microbiome, you can find out. The American Gut project in the U.S. is assembling a knowledge bank of bacteria that reside in participating individuals. For a fee, they will send you a kit and instructions for how to take swabs of bacteria from your body and mail them in to be analyzed. You then receive the results, indicating how your microbiome compares to others. The data may tell you if you have more or fewer Firmicutes in your colon, as well as other harmful and helpful bacteria. If you find you have a microbiome potentially tilted toward weight gain, what can you do to tilt it toward a lean one?

First, you can change your diet to contain more plant fiber that is challenging to digest—meaning fruits and vegetables—and fewer saturated fats. Not only does this reduce calories but also as your diet evolves, so will your bacteria. In experiments, mice that are fed a higher-calorie "Western diet" for eight weeks display higher levels of Firmicutes. But a diet including a healthy amount of fruits and vegetables and low in saturated fats allows the growth of diverse bacteria associated with lower weight.

Dr. Patrice Cani, of the Université catholique de Louvain in Belgium, studies the effect of prebiotics and probiotics on the microbiome. (Prebiotics are nondigestible plant carbohydrates that nourish the essential bacteria in our gut. Probiotics are actual bacteria that provide benefits to our health.) Cani says, "Prebiotics reduce food intake, and increase satiety in healthy subjects. They will change the composition or activity of some microbes, and will have a beneficial impact on health."

Cani's studies show that eating at least sixteen grams of prebiotics, contained in foods such as bananas, artichokes, and legumes, daily for two weeks promotes satiety and reduces eating. Oligofructose, found in onions, oats, and leeks, has also shown to effect a modest decrease in visceral fat mass, and decrease hunger. These prebiotic foods not only reduce appetite but also increase calcium absorption and are associated with greater diversity of bacteria in the gut, which is beneficial for weight loss. Prebiotics help induce a higher preponderance of Bacteroidetes, as well as a hundred-fold increase in another beneficial bacteria, *Akkermansia muciniphila*.

Cani has shown that *A. muciniphila* helps restores the mucous gut barrier that can be disrupted by a high-fat diet. Having a healthy mucous lining in our intestines creates a protective barrier, promotes healthy bacterial growth, increases innate immunity, and reduces the amount of toxins absorbed into the body. Ultimately, all this improves metabolism, lowers inflammation and insulin resistance, and helps reverse fat gain. Cani says, "High fat diets change the microbiota composition. If you change the microbiota composition, then in turn you can change gut biofunction."

Indeed, the microbiome is an exciting new field of research and, one day, if we can get over the "yuck" factor, we may even want to consider fecal transplants to import helpful bacteria. It's not too far-fetched—such transplants have been used to treat digestive diseases such as *Clostridium difficile* infection. In these experiments, a healthy donor's stool is transferred to the sick person, via an enema or endoscope, to replenish the patient's healthy bacteria in the colon and restore balance. After transplantation, the flora in patients' guts has been shown to be similar to that of the donor and their symptoms resolve with results that are even better than standard antibiotic treatment. Who knows? Fecal transplants for weight control may one day be coming to a clinic near you.

Chapter 7

I Blame My Parents— Genes in Obesity

We have all come to accept that our genes determine everything from the color of our eyes to the straightness of our teeth to our height, our talents, even our moods. But strangely, when it comes to fat, we tend to underestimate the effect of genetics. For the most part, fat is considered a personal failing—a punishment for lack of willpower, for eating too much, and for being too lazy to exercise and burn off those calories. We do tend to attribute the location of fat to genetic inheritance—as in, "Well, she got her mother's legs." And if we happen to be thin, we tend to credit that to a parent's genes as well. If we are overweight, however, it is usually considered to be our own doing.

Fortunately, science has come to the rescue by showing the many ways genes influence fat. This avenue of research is still new, since we have only recently begun to decode the mysteries of the human genome, but new studies are emerging every year.

A good example of how our genes can determine fatness is the story of the Pima Indians who crossed the Bering Strait from northern Asia and settled in the Americas approximately thirty thousand years ago. One population of the tribe settled near the Gila River in Phoenix, Arizona, and another kept migrating south, making their home in Maycoba, Mexico. The Pima sustained themselves by tilling dry soil to grow squash, corn, beans, and cotton, and by hunting small animals and other game. This lifestyle provided them a natural, well-balanced diet, and required them to get plenty of exercise.

What worked against the Pima, however, was drought, which occurred several times per century, destroying crops and reducing animal populations. Famine would follow and only those who could withstand long bouts of hunger managed to survive. The Pima endured these conditions for millennia, and geneticists believe that over time their bodies evolved a "thrifty genotype"—a set of genes that enabled them to subsist on very few calories by increasing the efficiency of their metabolism and storing as much energy as possible as fat. For centuries, this genetic adaptation helped to maintain the population. Then, during the mid-nineteenth century, the two Pima settlements started to diverge, with fascinating consequences.

The Arizona Pima started encountering Caucasian migrants in 1850 as they made their way to California in search of gold. The Pima assisted the weary travelers, offering food and protection. The outsiders, feeling welcomed, started staking claims along the Gila River, on which the Pima depended to irrigate their farms. With the ongoing gold rush in California, more settlers arrived, and the new farmers and ranchers started diverting water and land from the Pima.

Tensions arose, eventually leading the U.S. government to resettle the Indians on a reservation, though the Pimas' new land didn't include surrounding hunting lands or water rights to the Gila River. Without sufficient water for their farms, the Pima faced starvation.

The government offered food assistance starting as early as the 1930s. It included Western foods such as milk, bacon, cheese, canned meats, dry cereal; as well as flour and lard that the Pima used to make deep-fried bread. The lives of the Indians no longer included farming or hunting and they became more sedentary. Some Pima started to work in nearby factories, and others joined the armed services. Increasingly, they were introduced to the American lifestyle, and the Arizona Pima started gaining weight—lots of it.

The encroaching obesity among the Pima was noticed by the National Institute of Diabetes and Digestive and Kidney Diseases (NIDDK) in 1963 while they were doing an area survey. The rate of obesity and diabetes in the Arizona Pima was so high that the institute established research programs focused on the tribe to understand why.

The institute measured the health of the Arizona Pima every two years. Since 1965, tribe members have voluntarily undergone physical examinations specifically looking at weight, height, BMI, and factors for diabetes. The population of overweight Pima Indians was found to be more than three times higher than the U.S. national rate. The Pima also had drastically higher rates of diabetes. Yet Caucasians living nearby led a similar lifestyle without the same ill effects.

The NIDDK researchers also became aware of the Pima who lived in Maycoba, Mexico. As they were genetically similar to the Arizona Indians, the researchers wanted to know if both groups had the same health problems.

Dr. Eric Ravussin, of the Pennington Biomedical Research Center, based in Baton Rouge, Louisiana, was one of the first scientists to make the trek to Maycoba, high in the Sierra Madre mountains. Dr. Ravussin remembers, "There were no paved roads. There was nothing there—no electricity, no running water, nothing. No one had cars." It took researchers eight to ten hours using a four-wheel-drive vehicle through the rocky terrain to get to the village. The Maycoba Indians still farmed and rode bicycles in lieu of driving cars. For the most part they largely maintained the rural lifestyle followed by the ancestral Pima.

The Maycoba Indians were by far healthier than their Arizona counterparts. The Arizona Pima obesity rate was ten times greater among the men, and three times for the women; diabetes was five and a half times higher among the Pima of Arizona than for those in Maycoba. Clearly, the newly modernized lifestyle of the Arizona Pimas was taking its toll.

The tale of the two Indian tribes illustrates the genetics of fat at work. The Pima would not have survived the frequent famines through the centuries without evolving their thrifty genotype. However, in the time of plenty their genes are a liability, leading to high rates of obesity and diabetes compared to other races.

Eric Ravussin says, "I think that there is no question that these people, the Pima Indians, are at much, much higher liability when it comes to the impact of the changing environment on their weight, body fat, and glucose metabolism. It's about the interaction between their genes and their environment."

Eventually, analysis of DNA from the Pima suggested that they have variations on certain chromosomes that are linked to fatness. Thanks to their genetic inheritance, the Pima's bodies are storing away calories, anticipating a famine that never comes.

We can't change our genes, but science is learning that we can influence how they affect our health. And, as the Pima prove, there may be extra measures we need to adopt to accommodate our genetic peculiarities when it comes to fat. If we can't lose all the excess weight we've stored, at least we can shed some of the guilt associated with it.

We Are Not All Created Equal
When It Comes to Fat

Dr. Claude Bouchard, of the Pennington Biomedical Research Center, conducted some of the first studies showing that genes affect fat. After getting his PhD in population genetics and physical anthropology in 1977 from the University of Texas at Austin, Bouchard returned to his native Quebec and started a laboratory at Laval University where he and his staff became interested in studying obesity. Bouchard, who has receding curly hair and a friendly face adorned with glasses, says, "There were overweight and obese people in our environment, and their proportion seemed to be growing. We were recruiting families for our studies, and some of those families who volunteered were pretty heavy." This observation triggered Bouchard's interest and he expanded his lab to include additional staff who shared his growing curiosity about this trend in obesity. He recalls, "Pretty soon we had as many as fifteen people in the lab working in the field of obesity and exercise biology."

Bouchard and his team executed two foundational studies that upended the understanding of genetics and weight between 1986 and 1990, before the human genome project was completed. The first study showed that our propensity to gain fat, and where the body stores it, are influenced by genetics. He says, in his French-Canadian accent, "I was looking for an experimental model, in which we could manipulate body weight and truly test whether there was a genetic component to the variability in response. And I finally came up with a design based on pairs of identical twins. Using twins allowed us to contrast the response to diet or exercise of participants who are genetically identical versus those who are genetically unrelated."

Bouchard put twelve male identical-twin pairs on a diet of an extra 1,000 calories above their normal eating pattern for eighty-four days. As he expected, the young men put on a significant amount of weight—the average gain was 13 percent. Bouchard observed that twins were three times more likely to gain the same amount of total body weight, fat percentage, and subcutaneous fat than unrelated test subjects. Visceral fat was particularly correlated with genetics—it varied six times more between unrelated subjects than within a set of twins. In other words, if one twin gained visceral fat, then the other was six times more likely to also gain the same amount of belly fat than a nonrelative.

For a weight-loss experiment, Bouchard again isolated male identical twins in a research unit for four months. First, he measured the exact calories needed for the twins to remain weight stable at their current weights. He then imposed a standardized exercise routine of two hours per day, ultimately inducing a calorie deficit of 53,000 per person over the duration of the study.

As the twins slimmed down from exercise, Bouchard looked at body weight, lean mass, and fat distribution and found the amount of energy burned during exercise was also influenced by genetics. If one twin burned 80 calories compared to 100 burned by a comparator group during a workout, then the other twin would likely suffer the same metabolic shortcoming. He says, "The findings were again strong: about half the variation among people in their ability to successfully lose weight by exercise when caloric intake is kept at the same baseline level appears to be caused by genetic differences."

The pattern persisted across a variety of metrics. Bouchard found that our genes influence our resting metabolism, fat mass, percent of fat, and abdominal visceral fat, plasma triglyceride, and cholesterol levels.

Bouchard and his colleague Angelo Tremblay discovered one important exception, though—a vital piece of information for those seeking to control their weight. They found that when subjects performed vigorous exercise, genetics didn't matter as much. Bouchard's definition of "vigorous" was any exercise that caused metabolism to increase by six times or more over resting metabolism (which can be achieved by running about 4 to 6 mph or cycling about 12 to 16 mph, or doing other activities that produce rapid breathing and sweat within a few minutes). The lesson is clear: once we enter a specific range of strenuous exercise, the body kicks in to lose fat no matter what our genes want.

Bouchard's groundbreaking work tracing genetic aspects of fat in the 1980s and 1990s depended on observations of physical traits within families; statistical modeling to account for variables such as gender, age, energy intake and expenditure; and human experimentation confined to pairs of identical twins. But new technological advances are now allowing for more specific investigation of our genes. For example, individuals with variations in a gene called FTO tend to desire high-calorie foods more and have more fat as a result. This gene causes an almost twofold increased risk of obesity compared with those who do not inherit the gene variation.

One study that shows the effects of the FTO gene was conducted by Colin Palmer at the University of Dundee in Scotland. He assessed almost one hundred schoolchildren to see whether they carried the FTO variant gene or the normal FTO gene. He then evaluated what the children ate by allowing them to take food from a buffet that included an assortment of fruits and vegetables, as well as higher-calorie foods such as chips and chocolate. When he analyzed what they consumed, he noticed that children with the FTO gene variant had eaten more of the higher-calorie, energy-dense foods compared to children with the normal gene. Palmer says, "They had the same amount of food, the same mass of food, it was just the higher-calorie foods." Not surprisingly, children with the variant FTO gene also had about four pounds more body fat.

The FTO gene is thought to be expressed not only in the brain, where it increases our desire to eat fattening foods, but also in fat tissue. Harvard Medical School researcher Melina Claussnitzer and her team found that a single variation in the FTO gene caused fat cells that would normally become beige to turn into white fat cells instead. Beige fat cells, as described in chapter 1, have the potential to turn into energy-burning brown fat cells when activated by exercise. But in people with the FTO mutation, there are fewer cells turning into beige cells and more turning into energy-storing white cells. So the result of the FTO mutations is a drive to eat higher-calorie foods paired with less calorie burning, and more calorie hoarding. A challenging combination for any dieter.

Though individuals with variants in their FTO gene have almost double the risk of obesity compared with those who do not inherit the gene, Palmer explains, "Having the FTO variant doesn't mean one is destined to be fat. We can still control what goes in our mouths though it may be more work for some than others."

But not all fat caused by genetics is a bad thing. Some gene-related fat may actually be protective.

Ruth Loos is the director of the Genetics of Obesity and Related Metabolic Traits program at Mount Sinai in New York. She's slender, with short, wispy blond hair that frames her angular features. She has always been athletic, which led to her early interest in fitness. When Loos went to college in Belgium, she naturally decided to major in kinesiology and exercise.

Though Loos started out wanting to be a physical education teacher, the free education system in Belgium led her to other opportunities. She explains, "Belgium education is basically free. So you can hang around without creating debt. . . . I wanted to get a PhD, but I didn't really know in what. So one of my supervisors said, 'Go to the genetics department. We're doing this twin study, and we need someone to measure the twins—their height, their weight, their motor skills.' That's basically where I became an anthropometrist, where I really built the skill of measuring people— every part of their body."

Loos earned a master's degree in 1993 and a PhD in 2001 from the

University of Leuven in Belgium, and afterward received a grant to continue her research. The grant required that she study in an American lab. She knew of Claude Bouchard, who was by then at Pennington Biomedical Center, because he had written a textbook on physical activity and growth that she used in her master's program. She contacted Bouchard and soon became a postdoctoral fellow in his lab. Working with Bouchard, Loos grew fascinated with the genetics of fat and metabolism, and eventually went on to establish her own lab at Mount Sinai Hospital.

As Loos set out to design her research, she noticed that many genes being identified were linked to high BMI, which simply compares someone's weight to their height. Loos realized that BMI is not the best measure of fatness because it doesn't separate fat mass from lean tissue like muscle. In other words, if you are a body builder with only 7 percent fat but a lot of muscle, your BMI will be high, perhaps the same as that of someone who is obese with lower muscle mass. Loos wanted to tease out which sections of DNA had to do with fatness, not just weight. So her team conducted an analysis of the genetic data from 36,626 individuals to see which genes were associated with body fat.

From this research, Loos found that fatness was significantly linked to variations in the FTO gene and the IRS1 gene. It was already understood that variations in FTO were associated with being overweight, encouraging kids to seek fattier foods, for example. But the linkage of the IRS1 gene to fat was new. Loos, working with Tuomas Kilpeläinen and others on her team, quickly turned her attention to IRS1. As the team analyzed the data, they uncovered a mystery. One variation of the IRS1 gene caused lower fat in men. This at first seemed like a lucky gene to have. But as Loos analyzed the data further, she saw that while men with this variant indeed had less fat in their arms, legs, and trunk, they also had higher triglycerides and lower good cholesterol in their blood, and increased insulin resistance, all signs of ill health. How could this be? They were thinner than men without the variant, and thinness should lead to better health, not worse. More puzzling, this variant didn't seem to affect women in the same way.

Loos and team looked further. Perhaps this adverse metabolic profile was linked to how fat was distributed. Her team reviewed measurements for subcutaneous fat and visceral fat. They found that men with one IRS1 variant (call it variant A) had lower subcutaneous fat and a higher proportion of visceral fat, compared to those without the variation. In other words, even though they had less body fat overall, they had an unfavorable distribution of it.

Men with a different variant of IRS1 (call it variant B) had higher levels of subcutaneous fat, but, as Loos describes, "This variant that increased fatness was associated with reduced type 2 diabetes, cardiovascular disease, lower triglycerides, lower LDL, higher HDL, and so on." The men with variant B were fatter but also healthier.

Why would the gene that produces more fat protect you against disease? Loos wondered.

Slowly, she and her team were able to piece together an answer. IRS1 contains the code for a protein that is involved in mediating cells' sensitivity to insulin. She found that IRS1 variant A was associated with lower expression of this protein in subcutaneous fat and visceral fat. So, cells in these areas were not as sensitive to insulin, and were not internalizing glucose and fats. This occurred in men much more than in women.

In addition, IRS1 variant A was inhibiting adiponectin, which enables the expansion of fat tissue. With lower than normal adiponectin levels, men with variant A were not able to create new fat cells and expand their subcutaneous fat tissue. Their fat was hanging around in the blood, presumably depositing in their liver and pancreas, which was causing the increased dyslipidemia (elevated triglycerides and bad cholesterol, and reduced good cholesterol) and leading to insulin resistance.

On the other hand, those with IRS1 variant B had more of the IRS1 protein and more adiponectin. More adiponectin enabled easy expansion of fat tissue in the subcutaneous layer—that is, they were a little chubbier. For these men, their fat cells were internalizing sugars and fats, and keeping their bodies healthy. They had lower circulating triglycerides, cholesterol, and insulin levels.

Loos's findings were significant because they described a new kind of fat gene. Other gene variants—like mutations in FTO or the gene for leptin—had been linked to overeating or fat cell type. But IRS1 was the first that was linked specifically to fat cell creation. When we don't create new fat cells to house our circulating fats, we are prone to more diseases. With less fat, we may appear to be healthier, but may actually be in danger of developing diabetes and other diseases.

Loos says, "Genes that increase your risk of obesity can also protect you from type 2 diabetes, cardiovascular disease, and give you an optimal lipid profile. These are what we call the healthy obesity genes. So these individuals who had the variant to increase fatness actually were good fat storers. They store the fat where it should be stored. And it protects their liver, it protects their muscle, it protects against visceral fat. And that fat protects them against disease as well. So these [good] genes, they do exist."

Genes Are Strong, but Don't Have the Final Say

Just a few small changes in our DNA code can cause us to metabolize and distribute fat differently, and affect our behavior toward food. For some, more food will deposit as fat; for others, some food will linger in the blood and deposit in other areas. There will be people like the Pimas who gain weight easily, and others who can eat a mountain of food and not gain much.

You can undergo a diagnostic test to find out whether you have any known gene variants that are associated with obesity. If you have such a variant, are you doomed to a life of flabbiness?

The good news is that unless you have one of the very rare genetic mutations that undeniably cause obesity (such as the one that afflicted Layla Malik, described in chapter 2), your genes are just one factor in your weight profile. In the end, daily actions matter more. How much we decide to eat, what we eat, and how much we choose to exercise will, in the majority of cases, trump our genes. Fat genes like the FTO variant, however, make it harder to stay on track and keep weight down.

Loos explains, "You may be genetically susceptible to become obese, but it doesn't mean that you're destined to become obese, which is what many people think. They think, 'I can't do anything about it because it's in my genes.' The studies that we've done show that you may carry the obesity predisposing genes, but if you're physically active, or if you live a healthy lifestyle, you can reduce that genetic predisposition by 30 to 40 percent."

Loos's research shows that exercise is the key to combating our fat genes. In one study, she and her team collected information from about 218,000 carriers of the FTO gene and calculated that they had a 23 percent higher likelihood of being obese than those without it. However, some of those subjects engaged in regular physical activity, which significantly cut the odds of obesity for them. By being active, these individuals reduced the effect of FTO by 27 percent. This does, however, still leave about 70 percent of the fat-producing effects of the gene intact, but exercise at least helps temper obesity in those who are destined to struggle with their weight.

According to Loos, thirty minutes of physical activity at least five days a week may be enough to attenuate the effects of the FTO gene. She says, "It doesn't have to be overly vigorous as long as you start to sweat," which means even gardening, walking the dog, or riding a bike can work.

If you have a genetic predisposition for fat, nature will be working against you, and staying thin will be difficult. Your genes are not your fault, and it is easy to give in, but you don't have to. If you can muster Olympian self-control to substitute the energy-dense foods you're driven to with lower-calorie foods, and exercise daily, you can still control your fate. There is no doubt, though, that keeping poundage down will require by far more effort than it does for your peers without fat genes. As Loos puts it, "If you're genetically predisposed, it's going to be harder, but it's not that it cannot be done."

Chapter 8

I Am Woman,
I Have Fat

Martha Gray was a twenty-eight-year-old chemist when she met Tom in the lab where they worked. Martha had always been a bit nerdy and outspoken, which had turned off many young men in her past. But Tom, with his fiercely introverted nature, seemed to take her personality in stride, as if it filled a gap for him. After just six months of working together, Martha and Tom saw that they were the perfect combination of introvert meets extrovert. They got engaged, moved into an apartment together, and started preparing for a wedding.

Martha was not slim. She was five-foot-six, with short black hair and dark-rimmed glasses; she had been about twenty-five pounds overweight since her late teens. She was self-conscious about her appearance and decided to put off the big day by a year to give herself time to lose some pounds. She wanted to look like the brides in the magazines.

Martha had grown up as an only child, and her parents indulged her with all things girly—frilly bedding, dollhouses, and nice clothes. She was organized and prided herself on keeping her beautiful things tidy. As she settled into the new apartment with Tom, she started noticing how different everything was for this man. Tom tossed his clothes carelessly on the bed, threw his socks around the house, and left his toiletries messily near the sink. He had an established rhythm to his day, responding to e-mails in the morning, working by 8 a.m., watching TV at night, and reading in bed. He also liked to eat a certain way—a lot.

Tom ate constantly. He was thirty years old, six feet tall, and slim. He started his day with two bowls of cereal. Then he had a snack at 10 a.m., followed by lunch with lab mates, when he would typically order a foot-long sandwich. He broke for coffee around 3, and then ate a big plate of pasta or meat and potatoes for dinner. And right before bed, a large bowl of ice cream. Tom ran occasionally, but was not religious about it. To Martha, his sparse workouts did not account for how much he could eat without gaining an ounce.

And there was Martha who monitored every bite she ate, counting every calorie, struggling to make her wedding-dress dream come true. But she also wanted to be closer to her fiancé, so they regularly made large dinners together. And it was fun to share a bowl of ice cream at night and talk about the events of the day.

It remained fun until, after a few months of happy domesticity, Martha noticed that her pants no longer fit. She had gained fourteen pounds. Her thoughts ran rampant: "But I only added the ice cream. . . . He eats three times as much as me. . . . He doesn't even watch his weight and he's as thin as he was in high school. . . . It is not fair." Martha ate significantly less than Tom and yet the fat on her butt and legs was far beyond anything Tom would ever have to endure. Now there were ten months until the wedding—she had less time to lose even more weight than when she started.

Why Women Get Fatter Than Men

It's true. Life is not fair. And neither is fat. Women have long complained that men can eat more than they do and not gain weight. I doubt there are many females in the world who have not been infuriated by this phenomenon. And now, science has proven that women are right. As usual. On all continents of the world, and in every race and culture, women store more fat than men do. Food intake alone does not account for the difference in fat retention. Both genders consume roughly the same percentage of fat as part of their diet—about a third of all calories—and men consume more calories overall than women at every BMI. But men and women process food differently, mostly because of genetics, hormones, and the biochemical pathways that cause food to be converted into fat (or not).

The difference between males and females can be observed as early as birth. Researchers at the University of Zaragoza in Spain reviewed fat measurements in over 4,500 newborns. They compared the measurements of their skin folds as well as their length and weight and noticed that in every instance the female had a thicker skin fold (more fat) than the male. Whether a baby was taller or shorter, a few days younger or older, lighter or heavier, the main thing that mattered when it came to fat was gender. Similar experiments done with thousands of babies in Ireland, France, Belgium and the United States all had the same conclusion. Even at birth, and possibly before, females are fatter than males.

Beginning at age ten, it gets worse. With the onset of puberty, subcutaneous fat increases significantly in girls compared to boys. By age seventeen, girls have anywhere from 44 to 93 percent more fat than boys. During puberty, girls gain fat at a rate of 2.2 pounds per year compared to boys, who gain only one-fifth that amount, though boys are heavier overall due to higher amounts of lean mass—muscle and bone.

Dr. Michael Jensen is a physician at the Mayo Clinic in Rochester, Minnesota, who has been studying the differences in fat storage between men and women for decades. He says, "When young girls and boys go through puberty, girls actually gain fat, and they redistribute fat in the typical feminine fat distribution. Men lose a lot of their subcutaneous fat." Meaning these gender-induced weight changes cause us to look more "male" or "female."

The National Health and Nutrition Examination Survey (NHANES), administered by the Centers for Disease Control, collected data on 15,912 subjects and showed that women of all descriptions—Caucasian, Mexican-American, or African-American—store fat more effectively than men. They showed that men consume 51 percent more calories overall than women. Though a likely explanation would be that men have more fat-free mass (muscle, bone, etc.) than women and therefore need more calories, when the average fat-free mass in men was measured it was only 33 percent higher compared with that in women. Men can thus eat more than women pound for pound and not gain weight.

Why are women destined to be fatter? Again, the answer lies in hormones and biology. There are obvious evolutionary advantages to having more fat. Fat tells our bodies that all is right in the world, there is enough food available for us to start puberty and bear children. As we've seen in chapter 3, menstruation and pregnancy will not even occur if we don't have enough body fat.

Once menstruation begins, fat levels will even fluctuate during each cycle, with dips in estrogen and a peak in progesterone causing changes in appetite and fat storage. Women crave fats and carbohydrates during the second half of the menstrual cycle, when estrogen levels decrease. In addition to cravings, the simultaneous peak in progesterone promotes fat storage by clearing the blood of triglycerides and storing them in fat tissue. It is believed that this clearance leads to the desire for fatty foods because the blood is devoid of this nutrient. So it goes, month after month—first cravings, then fat. It's a wonder anyone can lose a pound.

And when women do become pregnant, their bodies add still more fat. The weight gain occurs even when their caloric intake is unchanged, and sometimes decreased. Women accumulate anywhere from five to thirteen pounds of fat in pregnancy, even if they are undernourished. The weight gain is not happening by the slowing of metabolism—total energy expenditure goes up when women carry a child. Part of the explanation may have to do with bacteria, our tiny friends in the gut.

Ruth Ley and her team at Cornell University who transplanted microbiota from pregnant women into germ-free mice (see chapter 6) found that mice with bacteria transplanted from women in the third trimester of pregnancy got much fatter than the mice with bacteria of women in the first trimester. They found the microbiota composition changes profoundly during the gestational period, which may explain some of the gain—women's bacteria increase absorption of food during pregnancy.

However fat gets accumulated during pregnancy, thankfully a portion of it is converted to milk to feed the newborn. Indeed, breast-feeding allows rapid weight loss after pregnancy for many. That women use their body fat to make all-important breast milk underscores the biological necessity of female fat: the survival of the human race depends on it.

Another reason women store more fat than men is a process called "nutrient partitioning," by which the body stores some of the calories ingested as fat, and uses the rest for other purposes such as for immediate energy or for glycogen stores (see chapter 1). Depending on your body, you may consistently set aside more or less of your food intake for fat storage.

To revisit the bank analogy from chapter 1, partitioning is like getting a paycheck for $100 every week, and automatically diverting $20 of it into a forced savings plan such as a 401k. If the $80 that's left isn't enough to cover your bills, you have to find another source of income, because the $20 will go into your 401k no matter what. In body terms, if you haven't consumed enough calories to fuel yourself after partitioning some as fat, you will feel driven to eat more. Scientists have not yet uncovered a way to significantly alter nutrient partitioning, which means that even when we do manage to eat less, our biology may urge our appetite on.

Michael Jensen explains, "When it comes to excess energy intake, woman and men respond very differently. Women seem to do a better job at partitioning circulating fatty acids into subcutaneous fat than do men."

Men partition calories to fat, too, but at a lower level than women. The difference alone can add up to pounds of extra fat per year for women. Anthony O'Sullivan, head of the Department of Endocrinology at the St. George & Sutherland Clinical School, University of New South Wales in Australia, has researched the differences in fat storage between women and men. He says, "You really only have to change your efficiency of fat metabolism by just one or two percent. Our bodies consume and metabolize so much fat and we generally burn much of it up. So you've only got to be a little bit more efficient to actually gain fat." And apparently women are in this regard, as in so many others, more efficient than men, to our eternal torment!

Even among women, however, there is inequality. For example, Asians have more fat at any BMI compared to Caucasian women. African-American women tend to have less visceral fat but more subcutaneous fat than Caucasian women. This may be, as researchers have found, because Caucasian women can more easily switch metabolism to fat burning than African-American women after eating a high-fat meal. So ethnicity as well as gender influences our fat.

Fasting and Exercise— A Short-Term Advantage

Though women store fat more readily than men, they also use it more when energy is needed. Michael Jensen examined free fatty acids in blood after an overnight fast. He noticed that women were releasing 40 percent more fatty acids into their bloodstream than men to serve the body's energy needs. But at the same time, women were also able to store those fatty acids into fat tissue much more quickly after waking. In fact, women stored two to three times more fat per unit of tissue then men did. So although women burn fat more readily during times of energy need, their bodies are also very quick to create fat by storing circulating fatty acids.

Women also burn more fat than men during prolonged exercise. It appears that women's bodies are designed to reach for fat more quickly during exercise, while men burn more carbohydrate and protein. In studies, when men were given estrogen, the opposite occurred—they decreased their carbohydrate and protein metabolism during exercise and increased their use of fat.

This is good news, right? Not exactly. Before women race to the treadmill, they should know that nature has another trick designed to keep them fat. After exercise they tend to eat more than men do. Jensen says, "Men and women respond differently to physical activity. Men are imperfect at compensating for extra calories burned with physical activity, whereas women on average are very good at compensating for physical activity. Given access to generous amounts of nutrients, women will compensate better [eat more] than men." He calls it a "fundamental, built-in" response.

There is, of course, a biological explanation for calorie overcompensation. Researchers from the University of Massachusetts in Amherst studied a group of overweight, mostly sedentary men and women. They put them on a four-day exercise program and then tested their blood for changes, most notably in ghrelin, the hunger-causing hormone. They found that in the men ghrelin levels did not change much after exercise. But in women, levels jumped by a third. And when researchers added more food to the women's diet to compensate for the exercise, their ghrelin levels still remained 25 percent higher than before they started.

"It appears that when the energy level of exercise goes up, women eat more whereas men don't," says Dr. Joseph Donnelly, who studies obesity and the effects of exercise at the University of Kansas. "In our experiment, when both genders burn 400 calories, no one is really eating more. But it was obvious at 600 calories that women did eat more but the men did not. At higher levels of expenditure, women compensate for calories burned." Donnelly's research leads to a counterintuitive conclusion: women who burn more than 400 calories during exercise may get less return on that extra investment than expected due to a greater urge to eat.

Women also face another imbalance with men regarding the effectiveness of their workout. Anthony O'Sullivan says, "It's well documented that women burn more fat than men during exercise. You would expect that women should more efficiently lose body fat following exercise than men, but they don't. It's the opposite. If a woman and a man are exercising one hour a day, during the one hour the woman is going to be burning more fat than the male. In the other 23 hours of that day the woman is going be burning less fat proportionally than the male." Jensen acknowledges the greater calorie-burning ability of lean mass in men, "The normal-weight woman on average has about 30 percent body fat. And a man of the exact same height, weight, age is going to have about 15 percent body fat. So what that means [is] they're burning more calories just doing nothing."

Women are thus subject to two factors: they experience greater appetite stimulation and more efficient fat storage. "You can't just look at that one hour of exercise," O'Sullivan says. Women have more body fat, and they actually use that available fat, but "once that exercise is finished, they revert very quickly to more efficient ways to . . . store fat." In other words, women will naturally tend to eat more after working out, and the food will turn to fat more quickly." So in the end, for women there is less fat loss from exercise than may be expected.

Maddening.

There is an upside to all of this efficient fat storage for women. Jensen explains, "The good thing about partitioning for women is that it keeps their lipids in the blood low. So their cardiovascular risk factors of high blood lipids are lower. It's healthier. The thing to tell men is you may be lean when you're young, but if you start gaining weight as you get older you're going to be in a lot worse shape than your wife, who might gain similar weight, because her adipose tissue is much more protective than a man's."

So, women's fat may actually be keeping them alive longer. Finally, a benefit!

Gender and Fat Distribution

Gender affects not just how much fat we have, but also where our fat is distributed. Testosterone and estrogen circulate through our bloodstream and bind to fat tissue. As our hormone levels change with age, pregnancy, exercise, or other life events, fat adjusts itself to the changing hormonal landscape and settles in different places accordingly.

As women might expect, estrogen causes the preferential distribution of fat to the thighs and butt, causing the bottom-heavy pear shape that is the fate of many females, whereas testosterone sends it to the belly, bestowing the typically male round-apple gut. Genetics also influences how our bodies interact with hormones and ultimately where we store our fat.

The effects of sex hormones on fat are so powerful that when men are given estrogen, as in the case of transsexuals, they gain body fat overall, even though their caloric intake is the same as before. Not only do they gain fat but they gain it disproportionately in the same places as women—the thighs and buttocks. The same works in the reverse—women-to-men transsexuals taking androgens (male hormones) lose fat in the hips, buttocks, and thighs and gain it disproportionately in the belly. Even small changes in hormone distribution can cause dramatically different effects on our fat.

Yet again, women can take some solace from this fact of hormonal life. Visceral fat of the kind men exhibit is more dangerous to health than the subcutaneous fat that women get on the butt and thighs. That's because fat under the stomach wall can surround the liver, digestive tract, and other internal organs and impede their function. It is also more prone to inflammation. The female fat stored just under the skin merely makes us . . . fat.

As women age, their estrogen levels decline, which you might expect would give them a break from all that hormonal fattening up. But you'd be wrong. At menopause, women gain even more fat overall, and adapt "male pattern" fat, too. Their bellies get bigger and contain more unhealthy visceral fat. They actually become a combination of pear- *and* apple-shaped, which sounds impossible but apparently is not. One study showed that postmenopausal women carry on average 49 percent more intraabdominal (visceral) fat than do women who have not yet undergone menopause. Women's fat-storage machinery actually works harder after menopause, meaning women utilize less fat and store more. Part of the reason is that fat tissue produces estrogen, which may explain why the body holds onto fat postmenopause. As men age, they too distribute fat differently, with excess going not just to the belly but also to the lower back and nape of the neck.

Neck fat! At least a small measure of justice.

Given all this, it is probably not a surprise that losing weight is more difficult for women than it is for men. Women eat less, yet gain proportionately more fat than men. And women must reduce calories more than a man would in order to lose the same amount of weight. This is not exactly news to women who have struggled for years with their weight, while the men around them ate abundantly.

What It Takes to Be as Lean as a Man

Of course, not every woman is content to accept her fate, fat-wise. Some are willing to take extreme measures, like Sherry Winslow, for instance. Sherry is fit and attractive, with angular features and shoulder-length blonde hair. She competed in body-building competitions from age thirty until forty. The average female body fat percentage is between 25 and 31 percent. Sherry maintained a training-weight percentage of around 15 percent. How did she do it?

At the peak of her career, Sherry trained for almost three hours daily, six days a week, paying a trainer $200 a week to oversee a gauntlet of challenging exercises. Training started at 5:30 a.m. Monday, Wednesday, and Friday and continued in the evening on Tuesday, Thursday, and Saturday, so that she could work around her day job. Her daily workouts consisted of an hour of hard cardio and ninety minutes of intensive weight lifting: abs, curls, squats, and bench, shoulder, and leg presses. Her trainer worked her hard and she pushed through until her muscles went limp. Every session left her drenched in sweat and completely spent. It was exciting, though, to see her muscles grow and stand out beneath her skin.

Sherry needed to get her body fat down to a very low level in order for her muscles to be visible to the judges of the competitions. At the same time, she needed to build significant muscle mass. This required enough nutrition to feed her growing muscles, but few enough calories that she could burn fat. A large percentage of her life went to planning meals and eating times.

After hours of hard workouts and doing her day job, Sherry would spend her nights shopping and cooking. Usually she made a few filets of fish or lean meat, brown rice, and steamed vegetables that she would apportion into five separate containers for her equally spaced meals the next day. Eating just enough at a meal to satisfy her hunger helped prevent excess calories from turning into fat. Cooking her own food helped her eat "clean," meaning none of the extra oils, heavy sauces, or unhealthy ingredients that customarily come with prepared food. To her lean diet she added nutritional supplements, protein shakes and vitamins to make sure her body had everything it needed to remain healthy. This specific regimen required a lot of work, but coming home at night and flexing her new muscles in the mirror made it feel worthwhile.

After a year of intensive training, Sherry was at 14 percent body fat and ready to compete. She bought spray tan, a shiny bikini, four-and-a-half-inch heels, and body oil to look her best. On stage, nerves nearly overtook her, and she started trembling. Being scantily clad in front of a full auditorium didn't help. But about halfway through her posing routine, she started to get excited. "I realized it's actually fun to be on stage at that point because you've done all the hard work," she says. "There's nothing more to do except pose, smile, show your personality, and let the judges do their thing." Sherry won her division, and went on to win the whole competition. "I felt a huge sense of success," she says. "It was like mission accomplished!"

Sherry has retired from competition now and works in San Diego as a personal trainer and nutrition coach. She doesn't generally recommend her training regimen to her clients, and instead works with them to find a weight-control strategy acceptable for their lives and bodies. "Setting a realistic goal is very important," she says. "Fat loss can be easier for some body types than others. You should learn which type is yours and set your expectations and fitness program based on the body type." Sherry admits that as a woman getting to 14 percent body fat was an all-consuming endeavor. It left little time for anything else. Thankfully, she does not expect her female clients to match that goal!

He Said, She Said

Nature has designed women to have more fat than men, but does this mean that they have to be overweight? No. But it does mean that women cannot match men 1 for 1, or perhaps even ½ to 1, when it comes to caloric intake. Though diet and exercise may not produce the same fast results that men get, understanding the reasons for the differences hopefully will empower women to stay with their diets and not get discouraged.

In addition to addressing physiological differences between men and women, the psychological differences are also important to consider. Many weight-loss practitioners comment on the difference in attitudes between the men and women they see. Sherry Winslow says, "My male clients can be much more intense in their pursuit of weight loss. They'll often make bets with their friends or make losing weight a competition of its own. They come to me more because they want to be better at sports or compete in some way. Women have more challenges they deal with every day. Many of my female clients are the main caretaker of their families and put others ahead of themselves. They're around food all day, they'll cook what their kids want to eat, and sit down for the meal with them, they'll shop for what the family wants to eat. Women need to carve out their own space to focus on themselves." Keeping in shape requires a selfish effort.

Another fundamental difference Winslow notices is how unforgiving women can be toward themselves. She says, "If women make one mistake and go off their diet, that leads to laxness on another decision, and another. With one transgression, they seem more likely to give up and just go off the diet all together. My male clients may have a beer the night before and they say, 'So what, I had a beer' and get back on the program." Sherry adds counseling and pep talks to keep women on track.

Indeed, research on fifty-four women showed one of the biggest failures for long-term weight loss is dichotomous thinking— meaning the tendency to make everything black or white instead of perceiving increments. It includes thoughts such as, "If I don't get an 'A' grade, then I failed." Dieters with dichotomous thinking have thoughts like "I broke down and had ice cream. I've failed at my diet and I don't see much point of going on," rather than, "I had ice cream but now I'll just continue on my diet."

Dichotomous thinkers tend to be less satisfied with themselves initially, and believe their weight loss is inadequate. This negativity just compounds dieting obstacles and leads to early abandonment of the plan. Such attitudes were significantly higher in women who regained weight after initial weight loss in the study. This attitude is not only bad for weight management, it can also lead to depression, eating disorders, and an inability to handle stress.

Michael Jensen says, "What I observe in my clinical practice is that when I'm counseling or working with women around issues of food, it's a much more personal, emotional issue than it is for guys. For guys, if they're eating too much, they're just eating it. They say, 'It just tastes good, so I eat more, Doc.' For women it has to do with comfort, and relieving stress, and all these kinds of things where they're getting something out of food that guys aren't on average." To work around this issue, Jensen gets input from behavior specialists who present cognitive restructuring to help women find relief from something other than food. Jensen says, "Behavior therapy is very important to bring in to the treatment of women, whereas for the guys it isn't typically as necessary. I tell women that I've got this really good behaviorist here that I'm going to refer you to, who can work with you for specific messages that hopefully are going to help you stop using food as your release. That helps with advancement pretty quickly."

Having meaningful goals can also determine whether or not women dieters succeed. It is not realistic or necessary to fit into the same bikini you wore in high school. Our bodies change with age, and once you've gained weight, your fat metabolism may be permanently altered, as studies by Leibel and Rosenbaum showed (see chapter 5). Picking smaller goals that are more attainable is a way to achieve incremental successes, which can encourage women to stay on the weight-loss path.

Choosing a goal that has true meaning is also important. Sherry Winslow says, "Many women tell me, 'I want to do this for my husband,' or 'I want to do this so I look better when I'm with my friends.' You have to do this for you. When there is a goal like 'I want to do this so I don't die,' it gives people more conviction to stay with the program." Indeed, as chapter 11 shows, pursuing weight loss to improve health is one of the strongest motivators for staying on a diet.

Alas, women should give themselves a break. Jensen says, "I always hear from my women patients, "My husband and I went on the same diet. He's down twenty pounds; I'm down ten. What's the deal?" Jensen encourages realistic goals, "Women have more well behaved fat. In other words, it's doing a better job of clearing fats out of the blood. If you're not really overweight, then you need to say just because the social convention is that I should have a BMI of 22, but I'm really 26.5, maybe I don't need to put all this effort in to lose weight. If one is healthy, that's the main thing."

The Wedding and Beyond

Throughout the year leading up to her wedding, Martha tried eating less and exercising more. But still the love handles remained. It seemed that no matter how hard she dieted, a bedtime dish of ice cream, even just once in a while, brought the pounds right back. After a year of struggle, she had lost just five pounds. Discouraged, she ordered a wedding gown two sizes larger than she had dreamed of and prepared to walk down the aisle. Tom was there to receive her. He met her the way she was and loved her that way. It was never about the pounds for him. Fifteen years after their wedding, Martha can smile. Once-skinny Tom now has a paunch. Maybe a little neck fat, too.

Chapter 9

Fat Can Listen

Ariana Green was an ambitious forty-five-year-old realtor in San Francisco. She was new to the business, which meant working seven days a week to build her reputation and client list. She was up for the challenge, though, and over time, her business grew. Ariana was also a beautiful woman who stood five feet ten and had blond hair, blue eyes, and high cheekbones. Her mother was a fashion model and Ariana inherited her good looks, which certainly had its advantages.

As Ariana marched through her late forties, she started gaining weight. At first she attributed this to the stresses and erratic eating habits that came with the new career. Then came a knee injury that slowed her down for a while. In the past, she'd always been able to shed weight easily. However, this time was different. Now fat appeared out of nowhere and seemed determined to stay. Her clothes became snug so she would go to a bigger size, and then it would happen again six months later. She was putting on weight like never before, and feeling depressed and confused about it. Finally, at fifty, something happened that shocked her: Ariana saw a snapshot of herself standing in the water in Cancun.

"I was absolutely obese," she says. "I hadn't realized it had gotten this far."

On a different continent but also in the same physical predicament was Mike Hanson, a forty-eight-year-old software engineer living in Sydney. His job was demanding and entailed traveling from Australia to northern California and China. Mike was no stranger to hard work. He had competed with Silicon Valley tech jocks for years and could hold his own. But now, in middle age, things seemed different. He was getting a spare tire around his waist and feeling sluggish. The punishing work schedule was bad enough, but when Mike turned fifty, his wife left him. His stress level shot through the roof. Suddenly, he was in a depression, and the spare tire was joined by fat elsewhere on his body.

What were Mike and Ariana doing wrong? They made the mistake of aging. With age comes hormone decline and stress, and our bodies change in many ways. Among the most frustrating is that we accumulate fat more easily, and lose it only with difficulty. Worst of all, fat begins to appear in new and strange locations that we never had to worry about before.

Different Age, Different Fat

Fat takes on different responsibilities at different ages. The younger we are, the better our fat behaves. When we are infants, a good proportion of our fat is the brown type, which burns calories and produces heat. At this stage, fat's primary functions are to keep us warm and safe as we leave the womb and enter an uncertain world. Babies have more brown fat, percentage-wise, than any other age group. Baby fat also serves to cushion us from falls and injuries. As we grow out of infancy, the proportion of brown fat decreases and white fat increases.

In our teenage years, fat changes function again and plays a key role in sexual maturation. It helps trigger puberty by telling the brain that we are sufficiently well fed to bring offspring into the world. Without the proper level of body fat, sexual development is delayed. As discussed in chapter 3, one way fat controls maturity is by secreting leptin, which aids in producing menstruation in girls. Another way fat regulates puberty is by producing estrogen, also critical for development. As their bodies get ready to bear children, girls will start to pack on more fat compared to boys.

Once the childbearing years arrive, it is baby fat, part two. Fat and the estrogen it produces are needed for women to get pregnant. Females must have the right amount of fat—not too much or too little. They will continue to gain fat in pregnancy, some of which will be used to produce milk for lactation. For nursing mothers, fat is used to foster the next generation.

Fat-wise, at this stage all seems right in the world. Then we hit middle age. And everything changes. As we approach our forties, production of the three sex hormones—estrogen, testosterone, and progesterone—which have heretofore been plentiful in our bodies, begins to wane. And, not coincidentally, our body fat suddenly becomes troublesome. It begins to shift from places where it once seemed so appealing to locations where it is anything but. In men, it now accumulates in the belly, the lower back, the nape of the neck. Women's fat settles in the belly, too, and on the thighs, buttocks, and breasts.

As we age, our fat mass peaks. Between fifty and sixty, we are typically at our heaviest and have the most difficult time keeping fat in check. Many people who were thin since childhood suddenly struggle with weight. "What is going on?" they ask.

Fat Has Ears

We know that fat can talk (chapter 2). It sends out messengers in the form of chemical signals like leptin to our brains, bones, and reproductive system. But just as fat can talk, it can also listen. This extraordinary property of fat was actually noticed decades before researchers knew it could talk.

In 1969, Dr. Pedro Cuatrecasas at the National Institutes of Health ran experiments in which he combined fat cells and insulin and noticed that the insulin made fat cells act differently. When insulin was present, fat cells would increase their conversion of glucose to fat.

Cuatrecasas refined his experiments to understand how insulin was having such an effect. After some searching, he determined that fat cells had receptors on their surface that were uniquely designed to bind to insulin. And once insulin was bound to a receptor, the behavior of fat cells would change to produce more fat. Receptors are like "ears" on the cell's surface that pick up incoming messages from the body. They are part of a two-way communication path whereby fat talks to the body (by emitting hormones such as leptin and adiponectin, as discussed in chapters 2 and 4), and the body talks back to fat (by sending hormones to fat). In the case of the insulin receptors on fat cells, these "ears" would "hear" insulin (coming from the pancreas) on the cell's surface and signal to fat cells to absorb more glucose and produce more fat.

Soon, other receptors were located as well. Dr. Thomas Burns at the University of Missouri School of Medicine and his team found that fat cells also had receptors that could bind adrenaline, which communicates to adipocytes to release fat into the system for energy. If you see a bear, adrenaline tells your fat: "Don't hoard energy for later. Use it now! Run!" Fat hears that signal and starts to release free fatty acids into the system for energy.

In the decades to come, it was discovered that fat has receptors for our most potent hormones—thyroid hormone, growth hormone, estrogen, testosterone, and progesterone. All these hormones tell fat when it is time to liquidate and release energy into the system.

When we are young, we have an abundance of these hormones. They work to grow our tissues, activate our reproductive systems, and keep our energy and metabolism high, which helps young people lose weight faster and keep it off more easily. But when we approach middle age we no longer need to activate our reproductive systems. Biologically speaking, we've outlived our usefulness. At this point, the production of most of those hormones decreases, which means the messages to our fat to dissolve itself are less powerful. With our bodies burning less adipose tissue through hormonal messaging, we inevitably get fatter.

At the same time, another hormone, cortisol, increases with stress and age. Cortisol is released from the adrenal glands in response to ongoing stress and is correlated with higher abdominal fat. All these hormonal changes together make it easier for fat to grow. We see it happen before our eyes; even though we may not be eating more than when we were young, fat now sticks to us more easily.

Women especially experience this weight gain as they approach menopause. During this period their hormone levels plunge as their ovaries head for retirement and produce less estrogen, progesterone, and testosterone. Lower estrogen levels cause increased appetite, reduced fat burning, and a redistribution of fat to the belly area, not to mention hot flashes and decreased energy. Furthermore, as the ovaries produce less estrogen, the body begins to rely more on fat's ability to manufacture the hormone. Fat becomes a dominant source of estrogen in postmenopausal women. It is hypothesized that this dependence is one reason women have a more challenging time reducing their fat compared to men.

Progesterone also declines significantly, altering the progesterone-to-estrogen ratio and causing a condition known as "estrogen dominance." This can lead to irritability, depression, sleep problems, water retention, a bigger appetite, and sugar cravings. It's like premenstrual syndrome, except that it lasts for years.

Testosterone, which is critical for both sexes, also decreases, causing a reduction in lean body mass and energy, ultimately leading to slower metabolism. Though we tend to think of testosterone as the male hormone, there is more of it in a woman's body than estrogen at most times of the month, and certainly during the perimenopausal or postmenopausal years.

Amplifying the Signal

The middle-age hormonal transition is what befell Ariana Green. That's when her fat came on fast and furious. She recalls, "I was slim for most of my life, maybe vacillating by ten or fifteen pounds here and there with a little bit of yo-yo dieting, but nothing of any great concern. And then all of a sudden I started putting on weight really rapidly."

Some of Ariana's gain was attributable to working long hours and not exercising enough. But those lifestyle issues were compounded by her changing hormones. The two factors together had a colossal effect. Ariana says, "When I turned fifty, all of a sudden I was gaining weight and having a lot of emotional trauma. I couldn't understand what was happening to me."

Ariana wasn't sure what to do, so she just soldiered on, building her career and quietly enduring her body's strange changes. She thought she was juggling it all as well as possible. Then came that fateful moment when she saw the picture of herself in a swimsuit.

Over the course of a few years, Ariana had gained more than one hundred pounds and now weighed 315. She would lose fifteen or twenty pounds through a variety of diets, but the weight would slowly creep back. After seeing the photo, though, Ariana knew she had to do something different. For a woman who had always been admired for her beauty, she never felt so undesirable in her life.

Still, she wasn't sure what she could do except start another sure-to-fail diet. Then a friend asked if she'd ever considered bioidentical hormones, which are synthetic hormones designed to be just like our own. It sounded extreme to Ariana, but at this point she was open to anything.

A physician tested her, Ariana recalls: "I was told that I had almost no hormones in my body, that they had completely left. And so, it wasn't unusual that I was displaying the symptoms of weight gain, emotional distress, crying, confusion, exhaustion." She had struggled, she said, "to the point where I thought I was mentally ill."

She realized that fighting obesity was going to be an enormous challenge. Managing her weight would not be a one-time fix, but a chronic condition requiring daily attention. Ariana says, "This physician was one of the first people who actually said to me this is something that you're going to have to deal with for the rest of your life. And that was a real eye-opening thing."

Ariana decided to try hormone replacement therapy (HRT). She first used human chorionic gonadotropin, which is found in placenta and is known to suppress appetite and move fat to more desirable areas of the body. She started losing weight quickly, about ten to fifteen pounds a month. Soon, she started replacement therapy for other hormones as well, including thyroid hormone, progesterone, testosterone, growth hormone stimulator, and estrogen. Her doctors designed a mix that restored her hormones to the levels of younger years.

The treatment helped Ariana curb her hunger, increase her metabolism, stabilize her psychological state, and make the best of her diet and exercise program. She lost one hundred pounds, a display of how powerful hormones are. In an interview, she said, "I am now just thirty pounds away from my goal. Hormone replacement is not something I'll do forever, but for now it works."

Aware that there might be a chemical fix for their misery, some menopausal women try taking birth-control pills to manage the symptoms of hormone decline. Anthony O'Sullivan, who researches metabolism at the St. George & Sutherland Clinical School, did studies comparing transdermal estrogen (delivered through the skin using a patch) to estrogen pills. He found that women who took pills had more fat storage than those who took it by patch. O'Sullivan saw that pill takers oxidized less fat after a meal and put on about four pounds of body fat during the study. It appears that when estrogen is taken by mouth, it gets absorbed by the gut, processed by the liver, and rereleased into the bloodstream. The body responds with a protein called sex hormone binding globulin (SHBG), which absorbs not only the extra estrogen but also the testosterone in the blood, lowering levels of both. This can ultimately lead to even more fat.

It's not just women who feel the effects of hormones. As noted above, both sexes produce testosterone and estrogen, the difference being that men have much more of the former than women do. Testosterone is important for everyone's weight management because it helps build and maintain muscle mass. It also burns fat and increases energy. As testosterone declines with age, the result is a loss of lean mass and muscle tone, lower mental energy and more visceral fat. When lean mass and muscle tone go, metabolism slows even further, since muscle burns more calories than fat does.

The relationship between fat and testosterone in men is circular— lower testosterone leads to an increase in fat, particularly belly fat; in turn, higher fat lowers testosterone. It is a downward cycle in which fat begets fat. And once you get into this cycle, it takes a lot of effort to get out.

Mike Hanson experienced the testosterone cycle firsthand. Like Ariana Green, age and stress in Mike's life combined in such a way that made weight gain easy. At the same time, his testosterone levels were declining naturally with age, making him even fatter. Mike knew he was in a low place. He recalls, "I was on traditional antide-pressants and I felt terrible. They made me gain weight, and I was lazy and unhappy." He found it much easier to get a quick burger and fries than to cook a healthy dinner, much less exercise every day. He knew he had to do something, but lacked the energy to climb out of his pit.

A friend suggested that Mike have his hormones checked. He found a specialist who thought that some rebalancing might help. Mike started on a testosterone stimulator and estrogen blocker. He says, "A big motivation was that I was fifty, I had very young chil-dren. I need to be alive for them when I'm in my seventies." Within about eight weeks after starting hormones, Mike felt the effects: "There was a change in how I thought about things, my concen-tration improved, my focus improved, and just generally felt more alive and awake." The boost of testosterone gave Mike more energy. He now had the motivation to exercise and cook a healthy dinner after work instead of watching TV and eating fast food. Mike says, "It's a virtuous cycle. I joined a yoga class four or five times a week. I started doing simple calisthenics exercises every day. I really focused on eating well." From a peak of 205 pounds, Mike brought his weight down to 160 pounds eighteen months after starting therapy. He stopped taking antidepressants and felt much better.

One surprising outcome of hormone therapy for Mike is that it made him appreciate the lives of women. He says, "When I took the testosterone booster, I was thinking, 'Oh, my God, I'm looking good. I'm feeling great. I'm working out. I'm feeling sexy.' And then some days I'd wake up and look in the mirror and say, 'Oh, my God, I'm looking fat.' I finally tied that experience to when I was due to take the estrogen blocker. Too much estrogen made me think I was fat. And I finally realized what my ex-wife and girlfriend go through when they say 'I'm feeling fat today.' It's like, wow! It's the estrogen, literally!" Mike was discovering that hormones affect our attitudes—how we view ourselves, and how we view others. Surely, Mike's girlfriend appreciates his newfound empathy!

Testosterone is perhaps the most potent fat burner we have. A study published in the *New England Journal of Medicine* showed that

even without any exercise at all, men who were given 600 mg of testosterone weekly for ten weeks built significantly more muscle mass
compared to those who were not administered any extra hormone.
The subjects built up more lean mass over the ten-week period than
men who did supervised strength-building exercises three times per
week but were not given testosterone. The study suggests that even at
rest, doing no exercise whatsoever, men can lose fat and gain muscle
thanks to an abundance of testosterone. Having copious amounts
of the hormone offers men a big advantage over women in terms of
weight management. But unfortunately for us all, testosterone production declines with age.

Another potent influence on weight that diminishes with age is
growth hormone, which is secreted by the pituitary gland. Growth
hormone is perhaps most well known for being present in children
and affecting their stature, but it also is involved in building lean tissue and burning fat in adults. As it declines, we tend to pack on fat.

To a lesser extent, thyroid hormone also ebbs in our later years.
This hormone produced by the thyroid gland affects metabolism and
body temperature. Production of it decreases more gradually than
growth hormone or the sex hormones, but for those diagnosed with
subclinical thyroid hormone weight control is more challenging.

Hormone Replacement Therapy in Perspective

So do we have to surrender to fat as we age? Not necessarily.
There are measures we can take to moderate our fat. One option is
to start hormone replacement therapy, as Ariana and Mike did.

Dr. Karron Power is a fit and energetic physician in San Francisco who prescribes HRT. She says, "What I found during my early
clinical years was that so many people were complaining about the
same thing. They were gaining weight, they were tired and didn't
feel good, they had less energy after work and had trouble sleeping.
They didn't have true depression, but were just feeling flat. I didn't
have the tools to help them. I could cover some of the symptoms, I
could give antidepressants or sleeping pills, but I really wasn't getting at the root cause of it."

Dr. Power entered a new field called antiaging medicine, a practice devoted to enabling people to live longer, and look and feel younger. HRT is one of the methods used. She explains, "It is the chicken and the egg syndrome. As people grow older, their testosterone and growth hormone levels decline. They begin to gain weight, which lowers these hormones even further, and continues the cycle of weight gain. Some doctors will tell patients that if they eat right, exercise, and lose weight then their testosterone and growth hormone levels will rise. It's partially true, but it can be hard to get people off of that spiral of decline. So we intervene—we get the hormones up." Power explains that with additional hormones, people start to feel better, they have more energy, which enables them to maintain an exercise program and invest more time in preparing healthy meals. The hormones also help reduce aches and pains after exercise and shorten recovery time, reducing barriers to regular exercise. She says, "With increased activity, natural hormone levels start to climb. If people continue to exercise and eat right, once they reach their goal weight they often can maintain success without further medical intervention."

HRT is not, however, without risks. Estrogen, even in its natural form, is linked to reproductive cancers in women, and can increase the risk of blood clots. In 2014, an FDA panel recommended limiting use of testosterone replacement products after data suggested increased cardiovascular events, such as heart attacks among men who were using them. Injecting growth hormone has also been associated with increased risk of diabetes. Clearly, HRT needs to be used with the guidance of a knowledgeable physician who can weigh the risks and benefits for any particular individual.

Mike Hanson also warns that with HRT "one of the problems is that you feel as if you can conquer the world. And one of the issues with that is that the rest of your body is not necessarily caught up yet. So it's very easy to over-exert yourself because you feel like you were when you were thirty. But you can't act like you did when you were thirty. I ended up actually tearing a muscle, which I wouldn't have done before the hormone stimulation program because I wouldn't have the energy to even think about crawling on monkey bars with a two-year-old on my shoulders. You have to do the stretching. You have to build up strength slowly."

Using HRT to slow the signs of aging is not widely embraced by the medical community at this time. Although women have been taking estrogen to offset the effects of menopause for decades, it will take years of study and persuasive data to fully characterize the risks and benefits of using hormone therapy to catalyze weight loss. In sum, HRT is a means of medical weight loss, similar to diet pills or surgery, with all the attendant risks and issues. Perhaps the best use of HRT is, as Power suggests, for a limited time to make it easier to get back on track, and then to revert to natural means of maintaining a healthier body.

Amplifying the Signal Naturally

Luckily, we can increase our hormone levels to some extent without a doctor. One of the natural ways to activate hormones is exercise. If we can overcome the sluggish feeling that weight gain causes and exercise at least three times per week for forty-five minutes, we can increase secretion of some hormones. Researcher Savvas Tokmakidis at Democritus University of Thrace in Greece had a group of men do a sequence of resistance exercises including four sets of eight squats and leg presses and saw that testosterone and growth hormone levels rose significantly afterward. Researchers Bradley Nindl and his team at the Military Performance Division in Massachusetts observed that a two-hour bout of aerobic exercise resulted in significant escalation of growth hormone for a twenty-hour period.

Exercise also increases adiponectin, the hormone emitted by fat tissue that moves fat away from the viscera to the limbs and hips. It improves insulin sensitivity, too, leading to lower blood glucose and triglyceride levels. The added benefit of most of these hormones is that they won't just burn fat, they'll increase lean tissue, which also leads to higher metabolism. So even at rest, we'll burn more calories.

The downside of exercise is that it may cause a hunger spike, which can lead to overcompensation at the dinner table. Karron Power advises her patients to start slowly: "People are often surprised when they try to exercise as hard as they can and I tell them to bring it down a bit. Intense aerobic exercise, say from running or a spin class, will burn calories but trigger appetite to such an extent that many will replace those hard lost calories, and then some. And weight training will increase muscle mass and resting metabolism—extremely important for weight maintenance—but it won't take off the pounds. I recommend walking an hour each day to burn extra calories without increasing appetite, with moderate weight training two to three times per week to increase lean muscle mass. Once they get a little more fit, then they can ramp it up."

What we eat and how much also affects our hormone levels. Our growth-hormone levels are naturally reduced by sugars and fats. That means eating a lot of cheesecake or other fatty desserts not only puts more fat into our bodies, but also diminishes our ability to burn it. It is a double penalty in which fat begets fat. Avoiding sugary foods also helps prevent the energy drop and hunger that result from insulin clearing the blood of nutrients. Eating about ten grams of protein after mild exercise, or twenty grams after more strenuous workouts, helps control hunger, as will adding plenty of fiber to one's diet.

Not eating anything also increases our levels of fat-burning hormones. Many body builders and work-out enthusiasts swear by intermittent fasting. When blood sugar becomes low, it triggers the release of fat-burning hormones including adrenaline and growth hormone. Growth-hormone release peaks at night and during sleep. Intermittent fasting is powerful partly because it prolongs the overnight fast, extending the release of growth hormone, which burns fat.

A common suggestion by trainers is a sixteen-hour daily fast (including sleep time) for women and a fourteen-hour fast for men. This means getting balanced nutrition within an eight- to ten-hour span each day, and letting the body go without food for the evening and overnight to extend growth-hormone release. Fasting also releases ghrelin (the hormone produced in the gut that stimulates hunger) which has been shown to further stimulate growth-hormone release. So prolonged hunger guarantees fat loss, but it does make fasting difficult.

Getting more sleep may also help. Research shows that lack of sleep increases ghrelin and lowers levels of leptin, the hormone that tells us we are full. Sleeping less than six hours per night has been shown to increase the risk of obesity, and is associated with lower insulin sensitivity, a precursor for diabetes. So without sufficient sleep you'll be hungry and less satiated all day, and eventually at risk for diabetes.

The Man Who Ate Plastic

Age, poor diet, and sleeplessness aren't the only disrupters of hormones. Environmental agents can also contribute. Xenoestrogens are chemicals in the environment that mimic the effects of estrogen. According to Dr. Power, ingesting xenoestrogens by mouth has the same effect as taking birth-control pills: the chemicals are absorbed through the gut and transported to the liver, causing an increase in sex hormone binding globulin, SHBG. This binding hormone not only absorbs the xenoestrogens, but potentially also the body's own testosterone. If we have lower testosterone levels in our systems, we are prone to gain weight.

Power says, "We know that there are a lot of endocrine disrupters in our environment. If I see signs of excess estrogen in a person's system that is blocking their testosterone, I talk to them about the four P's: Plastics, Preservatives, Produce, and Pesticides. Plastics often contain BPA and phthalates and cosmetic products often use the preservative paraben. Some plants, especially soy and flax seed, have high levels of natural plant estrogens, and nonorganic produce can contain man-made estrogen-like pesticides. I suggest replacing plastic with glass, buying products without paraben, eating organic foods, and limiting intake of soy and flax."

One of Power's patients felt the effects of xenoestrogens firsthand. Jerry was a very active forty-year-old who participated in a variety of sports, including water skiing and soccer. He was an adrenalin junkie and liked extreme activities such as bungee jumping and parachuting. One day he noticed he was putting on belly fat. He thought it was strange, because he hadn't changed anything in his diet or exercise routine. He ramped up his workouts, but his soft belly persisted. At the same time, Jerry noticed a change in his moods. He was losing motivation at work and, more importantly for him, losing motivation to bungee jump out of helicopters.

Dr. Power gave him a physical and examined his hormone levels. His production of testosterone, growth hormone, estrogen, and thyroid seemed to be in order—except for one thing: "His testosterone production was great, but his SHBG was very high, interfering with all that testosterone. As a result, he had early low testosterone symptoms. There was something else going on to cause high SHBG."

Power went through the list of xenoestrogens with Jerry. Using questionnaires and discussion, they were finally able to piece together the clues. Jerry had recently gotten married, and his new wife was cooking dinner every night. When she finished she would put the food into a plastic container while it was still hot, and then put it in the fridge to cool overnight. Jerry would take the container to work the next day and heat it in the microwave. Power says, "Heat can release xenoestrogens, like BPA and phthalate, from plastic and it can transfer into food. This new source of xenoestrogens was causing Jerry's SHBG to go up." The extra SHBG absorbed not only the estrogens but also the testosterone in his blood, causing Jerry's lack of energy and weight gain.

Power says, "I told him to switch from plastic to glass containers, and within a couple of months, his SHBG was down and his available testosterone was up. Nothing else changed. His actual testosterone production hadn't changed. But removing these plastics made those symptoms of low testosterone go away." Jerry's shift away from plastics helped him lose weight and regain his energy. He resumed his sports, started burning off calories, and is jumping out of helicopters once again.

Fat Is a Force of Nature

As both Ariana and Mike can attest, aging plays havoc on the waistline. Their biggest struggle was with hormones. As we age, the decline of fat-burning hormones and the increase in cortisol slows our metabolism, reduces lean tissue, makes us lethargic, and facilitates the accumulation of fat, particularly unhealthy belly fat. There are other issues too.

Exercise, for example, becomes less effective as we grow older. Dr. Paul Williams, a scientist at the Lawrence Berkeley National Laboratory, studied close to five thousand male runners aged eighteen to forty-nine, and found that no matter how many miles they ran, the older subjects gained weight. By the end of his study, he concluded that "waistline expansion is almost a force of nature," even in very active subjects. He found that men who exercise "will be leaner than sedentary individuals, but even devoted runners will find it increasingly difficult to remain sleek." Williams provides a ray of hope, however. "Our data suggests that you can probably compensate for middle-aged weight gain by becoming more active. By annually increasing weekly running distance by about 1.4 miles, we estimate that the effects of exercise should compensate for the expected weight gain during middle age. What this means is that runners who average 10 miles per week at age 30 should increase their weekly running distance to 24 miles by age 40 if they plan to still fit into the tuxedo they bought a decade earlier." Proof that with advancing age also comes advancing fat.

Fat listens to our bodies and responds in kind. Some messages tell fat to grow itself, while others suggest that it reduce its territory. Hormones provide very loud signals for fat, and they influence how much fat we have and where it will be located. Our bodies are programmed to lose hormones and gain fat as we hit our middle years, causing a shift in fat distribution.

But there is an upside to gaining fat as we age: it may protect us against mortality from disease. The obesity paradox, mentioned in chapter 3, shows us that for some age-related diseases, excess fat actually reduces mortality. Those with diabetes, heart attacks, and strokes have a lower death rate from their disease if they are overweight. The specific reasons for this are still unclear, but there is a chance that nature intended for us to get fatter as we age, as a cushion against death.

Moreover, the fat we gain in middle age isn't permanent. Surprisingly, once we reach our seventies, fat seems to go into reverse and we start to lose it. With age, fat cells shrink—they are no longer capable of holding as much fat. Though this loss of fat may seem like a final relief from our struggle with weight, it's not. Since our adipose tissue is less capable of storing fat, the molecules released from fat cells are forced to roam in our blood. Fat will start storing in some weird places, including bone marrow, liver, abdomen, and muscle tissue. This "ectopic" fat contributes to health problems such as weaker bones, decreased muscle strength, and higher risk of diabetes.

So, are we doomed to obesity and metabolic disease as we age? Not entirely. There are measures we can take to manage our fat. We need to exercise, eat wisely, and sleep enough if we are to gain some control over our weight. But even with that, managing fat will require more effort and discipline in middle age than ever before in our lives. Fortunately, for most of us, with age also comes wisdom and perspective—including the realization that a little extra fat here and there isn't such a big deal after all. The important thing is to be healthy, and if you are up for the challenge, you can keep your fat in line.

III

SO WHAT IS THE
SOLUTION?

Chapter 10

Fat Control I: How You Can Do It

We've covered a tremendous amount of information about fat— what it is, why it's important, the tools it uses to fight its demise, the unusual ways we gain it, and why it varies so much among us. Fat is complex. We love to hate it, but it's a critical organ that has more influence in our bodies than we think. Fat does its best to accommodate our needs, and in return it needs to be cared for just as any organ does. So now that we know so much about fat, what do we do? How do we minimize the dangerous visceral fat, and keep our beneficial fat at a healthy level?

Previous chapters show that the answer to those questions are as individual as anyone reading this book. Depending on your age, gender, genetics, microbiome, and dieting history, you may have either an easy or a difficult time managing your fat. Fat loss can differ significantly based on individual biology. For example, certain gene mutations can cause a strong desire for energy-rich foods and produce more white fat cells instead of beige cells (see chapter 7). If you have a history of gaining weight and losing it, even if that was five years ago, you are probably saddled with a lower metabolism and larger appetite than your thin, fit co-worker who never went on a diet (see chapter 5). Your age and changing hormones also impact how much you can eat and the extent of exercise you need to stay thin (see chapter 9). Infectious microbes you've come across may be influencing your weight in ways you never thought possible (see chapter 6). And if you are a woman . . . well, don't get me started (see chapter 8)!

Even the simple act of eating a muffin will have different consequences depending on your biology. Dr. Eran Segal at the Weizmann Institute of Science in Israel enrolled eight hundred volunteers to study their glucose levels after they ate various foods. He noticed that the same food would cause glucose to rise sharply in some but not in others. High glucose levels provoke insulin secretion, ultimately leading to more fat storage. Segal developed an algorithm that factored in each volunteer's genes, bacteria, and recently eaten meals and could actually predict which foods would cause a glucose spike. Sometimes foods on the plans were surprising—certain individuals could eat foods like chocolate or ice cream in moderation and not get a spike, while others couldn't. This research underscores the need to individualize diet plans.

And it's not only what goes into your mouth that's important to consider, but your psychology and lifestyle as well—what is tolerable for one person may be simply impossible for another. For example, there are diets that impose dozens of rules—specific ingredients to omit from your life and another list of foods that are imperative to eat in some specific quantity and schedule. Such complicated programs may work well if you have time to shop, cook, and create elaborate meal plans, but if you are a busy executive or parent, forget it. Most people need a simple but effective plan with foods that can be found anywhere. I've known personal trainers who prescribed two hours of exercise per day, five to seven small meals, and no sweets (no sweets?!). This regimen may be fine for a body builder, or someone who is self-employed, but for people like me with a full-time job and kids, it's not going to happen. I don't want to be eating in my office all day, smelling it up like a diner, and I can't be squeezing two hours out of every day to work out. Let's try for forty-five minutes a day of exercise instead.

There are so many well-intended diets out there, but they won't work if you can't stick to them. Your diet needs to be customized for you biologically, psychologically, and socially. Following someone else's plan may make you fatter instead of thinner, and can certainly make you more miserable. Don't be seduced by the siren song of losing weight easily if you just follow steps 1-2-3. It makes for easy selling of diet books, magazines, and TV shows, but may be a disaster for you. Pay attention to how your body reacts to food and exercise, and adjust accordingly. No one knows you better than you.

That said, there *are* well-researched, successful weight-control tactics that will work for many people. For every creative way that fat manages to reproduce itself, there is another way to offset it. If you truly understand fat, you can control it. Each chapter in section III provides solutions at the end to manage fitness pitfalls, and some strategies cut across many of the challenges. These approaches are summarized here.

Exercise to Address Genetics, Hormones, and Aging

Almost all of chapters in section II cite exercise as a means of reducing fat and keeping our bodies more youthful. As Claude Bouchard showed us (see chapter 7), genetics will cause exercise to have a greater effect for some people than others, but it is still one of the most powerful means we have to control our metabolism and weight. And at a certain intensity, exercise can even overpower a genetic predisposition to fat.

When we challenge our muscles, we signal to the body that we need more strength. Our bodies respond by diverting energy away from other tissues (such as fat) and toward bones and muscles. Strenuous activity builds lean body mass, which burns more calories, forcing fat to compete for resources with other growing tissues.

This is what happened with the sumo wrestlers described in chapter 4. They ate in abundance in order to be overweight, but as long as they exercised, they remained healthy. Remember the liposuction patients in chapter 5, who regained fat in the belly after having it sucked out of the buttocks? Patients who exercised regularly didn't gain back this visceral fat. If we are sedentary, fat will accumulate in areas near our internal organs and hurt us; exercise helps direct fat to the subcutaneous layer.

Exercise also promotes the release of adiponectin, growth hormone, adrenaline, and testosterone—all hormones that both enable fat to be used as energy and mobilize it away from the visceral area and into the periphery (see chapter 9). And exercise increases the body's sensitivity to insulin. This means our muscle and fat cells take up fats and glucose in our blood, preventing them from roaming around and harming other organs. Leptin sensitivity also goes up with physical activity, which increases metabolism.

With consistent exercise, the body starts making permanent changes. Eventually, the transcription of genes that build muscle and burn fat increases. With that shift, resting metabolism increases because muscles burn more calories than fat does. Exercise enhances key hormones and healthy fat, which is particularly important as we age and our hormone levels decrease. Exercise has even been shown to reduce the probability of other age-related maladies, such as dementia and weak bones. Another unanticipated benefit of exercise is that it produces more brown fat, which, as explained in chapter 1, actually burns calories instead of storing them.

The National Weight Control Registry (discussed in greater detail below) contains information from more than four thousand veteran dieters and confirms the necessity of exercise. According to data in this registry, only 10 percent succeeded by cutting calories alone. The rest incorporated diet and exercise in order to maintain weight loss.

Dr. Michael Dansinger, the physician who runs a successful weight-loss clinic at Tufts University (see chapter 4), says, "The main driver of weight loss is caloric reduction through dietary change. That is 80 percent. The other 20 percent comes from exercise. Without exercise, I get a lot of field goals, but not as many touchdowns. I might be able to get someone's diabetes two-thirds of the way to remission, but without the exercise I'm often not able to get someone all the way there."

The challenge that exercise presents is that it can cause a sharp increase in hunger that leads to overeating. Dansinger advises people to get a handle on eating before starting exercise: "In theory, you can offset all of your benefits of exercise just by eating too much after a workout. . . . Once someone's got a good handle on eating, we gradually aim for more exercise. Eventually I would like to see seven hours a week, two-thirds of it being cardio." Similarly, Dr. Karron Power recommends that her patients start off with walking. It eases them into exercise, and it's an activity they can increase gradually. If strong hunger pangs return, she advises them to reduce the exertion slightly until they are ready for more.

HIIT—A Power Workout in a Short time

We all have reasons for why we don't exercise. In addition to hunger pangs, time restraints are a common complaint. But that is no longer an excuse—High Intensity Interval Training, or HIIT, is a good way to get a vigorous workout in a short time—for example, four cycles of a thirty-second all-out sprint followed by a thirty-second low-intensity jog worked into a twenty-minute run. Another approach is twenty seconds of high-intensity activity and ten seconds of low intensity for eight cycles in four minutes worked into an exercise routine. HIIT workouts can provide the same benefits as traditional exercise, such as jogging, but in a shorter time. Plus, the research shows HIIT burns fat more effectively than steady-state exercise. So what's the catch? Only that HIIT is hard work and you must be prepared for a heart-thumping sweat.

If HIIT isn't for you, don't worry. Even those who engage in easier recreational activity like walking or casual backyard sports lose more weight than those who don't do anything.

Forty-Five Minutes a Day

Whether you include exercise from the beginning of your diet, or work it in later, it is a critical component of having healthy fat. Working out at least forty-five minutes a day, including thirty minutes of cardio and fifteen minutes or more of strength-building training, can do wonders for your health. Exercise helps us reduce dangerous fat, and make the fat that's left healthier. Even if you never develop six-pack abs, you can have healthy fat with enough activity.

Eating Effectively for Hormones

Depending on our genetics, gender, race, age, hormones, and microbiome, once we swallow food we each process it differently.

You may be able to eat as abundantly as a lumberjack, or you might have to eat as scantily as a monk.

We can't do much about our age, gender, or race, but science has shown us that food affects our hormones, and hormones affect our fat. Throughout this book you've seen how insulin, leptin, ghrelin, adiponectin, estrogen, testosterone, thyroid, and other hormones influence our weight. Our body is an intricate communication system and hormones are key players.

Insulin is an important hormone to manage. Overeating, as well as eating too many carbs, provokes insulin, which directs extra nutrients in the blood towards fat. Though some people can get away with eating high carbs, for many it is a diet killer. The best way to control insulin is to limit refined carbohydrates and balance complex carbohydrates with protein, fat, and fiber. Replacing some carbs with proteins will help to stave off hunger. Eating raw vegetables also allows us to eat more and keep our bellies full, which triggers stretch receptors in the gut. When stretch receptors are activated, they ultimately reduce ghrelin, the hunger hormone. Adding clear broth to a meal or in between meals will also add volume and stretch these receptors.

Leptin also needs to be managed. Ghrelin produces hunger and leptin satiates it. As we lose fat, our leptin levels will decrease, making us overall more hungry (see chapter 5). Additionally, there's evidence that shows diets high in fructose promote resistance to leptin. Staying away from high-fructose foods, particularly anything with high-fructose corn syrup, helps maintain a sensitivity to leptin. Getting adequate sleep also enhances leptin and keeps ghrelin low (see chapter 9).

Intermittent Fasting

Though hunger is uncomfortable, intermittent fasting has been known to work wonders, especially for hard-to-lose fat. Fasting not only reduces intake but triggers the release of fat-burning hormones including adrenalin and growth hormone. Most growth-hormone release happens at night and during sleep. Intermittent fasting is powerful partly because it prolongs the overnight fast, extending the release of growth hormone and thus the burning of fat. In addition, ghrelin, which makes us hungry, also enhances the release of growth hormone. So if you can stand the hunger, the longer you fast, the more fat you burn.

As mentioned in chapter 9, a common suggestion is a sixteen-hour daily fast for women and a fourteen-hour fast for men. Eating is limited to eight to ten hours during the day, and the fast spans the evening and night.

Mark Sisson, a former elite endurance athlete and well-known fitness educator, says, "I fast for eighteen hours per day. But rather than call it fasting, I call it my window of eating. I eat within a six- to seven-hour window, from about 1 to 7 p.m." Mark works out in the morning, before eating, with a routine that includes weight lifting and HIIT. He then waits until hunger really kicks in before he has lunch, his first meal. As an example of his diet, his 1 p.m. lunch on a certain day contained a piece of salmon on a bed of vegetables and just a little bit of rice. He snacked on a slice of cheese in the late afternoon. For dinner, he cooked up a steak and a side of vegetables and said he might have a little bit of chocolate afterward. This was his intake for the day—two main meals and a snack. He starts his fast in the early evening through to 1 p.m. the next day.

Though Sisson is a veteran of intermittent fasting, he admits that it does not work for everyone: "If you are a heavy carb eater and your body depends on carbs, fasting will be hard. You have to already be in fat-burning mode, which is done by reducing carbs and getting your body used to burning more fat. Once you are in that mode, you can prolong the fasting time. But if fasting makes you miserable, don't do it. Who wants to spend their lives being miserable? You have to do what works for you."

Sisson has benefited a great deal from his fasting program. At sixty-two he is muscular and fit and looks every bit like the Malibu surfer he is. He suggests a low-carb diet, and trying to miss one meal first, letting the body get used to the drop in nutrients, and then extending the interval between meals. Drinking plenty of water and broth helps ensure the right electrolytes. He adds, "Ask yourself if you are really hungry and whether you need to eat more. If you are no longer hungry, don't take another bite. Your body will get used to less eating." The key, he says, is to not overcompensate when you finally eat again, and to take in protein, fiber, and water to fill up.

Eating for the Microbiome

Depending on the distribution of bacteria in our microbiome, we may be extracting more or fewer calories from our food than other people, as explained in chapter 6. In turn, what we eat influences the composition of our microbiome, which then further affects our weight. Taking in more fruits and vegetables has been observed to reduce the proportion of energy-harvesting bacteria and also increase the overall diversity of bacteria, both of which are associated with leanness.

The main takeaway is that the more fibrous salads you have, the better. Eating more leafy greens and raw vegetables makes us fuller on fewer calories, helps diversify our bacteria colonies, reduces the relative population of energy-harvesting bacteria, and enables the growth of bacteria that pass more food on as waste. If you include in those salads ingredients that nourish a healthy microbiome, such as legumes and vegetables high in oligofructose like onions, leeks, and artichokes, then you are on your way to satiety with fewer calories accompanied by less calorie extraction (again, see chapter 6). So lower-calorie, higher-fiber foods lead to weight loss, and ultimately to a healthier microbiome that extracts fewer calories still. As we start to get thin, our bodies are primed to get even thinner, and in this way thin begets thin.

Food and Women

Women utilize and store fat differently than men, as described in chapter 8. Women burn more fat during exercise than men, but they also store it much more efficiently. And as Joseph Donnelly's studies show, women have a greater tendency to overeat after expending 600 calories or more from exercising compared to men. Therefore, while women should definitely exercise (they burn a lot of fat), they need to be very disciplined afterward. Donnelly did see that exercising off 400 calories didn't produce the same urge to eat afterward. One solution is to do more moderate exercise and stay below the 600-calorie limit. Another is for women to exercise to their heart's content, but use distraction methods to not overeat afterward—watching television, engaging in conversation, or running errands, or pursuing some other interest to turn their attention away from food for at least an hour. Most likely, that overpowering, I-just-worked-out urge to eat will go away.

These same distraction tricks can also help us avoid emotionally driven eating. Dr. Michael Jensen discussed how emotions play a larger role in overeating for women compared to men (see chapter 8). Counseling, willpower exercises (see chapter 11), and other forms of stress relief, such as jogging, going for a walk to get fresh air, or hitting a punching bag might be helpful here. Emotions and food interact in complex ways, and these suggestions may not work for everyone. But be creative—if you reach for food out of frustration, then what can you reach for in its place?

Curbing overeating is also important because women partition more nutrients into fat than men do. With partitioning, the body stores away some part of food in fat regardless of its immediate energy need. So even a small amount of food leads to more fat in women compared to men, and excess amounts of food will lead to even more (see chapter 8). Try eating slowly, allowing smaller meals to last longer and trigger satiation. Use discipline or distraction as a tool to not overeat—ever! Remember, salads and high-fiber foods that are filling and tend to pass as waste rather than being deposited give you an advantage.

As we have seen, the menstruation cycle in women also has specific consequences for fat (see chapter 8). We know the luteal phase of the menstrual period (second half of the month) promotes cravings and fat storage. Because of this, it is best to wait until this stage has passed to initiate a diet. Beginning any diet takes willpower and close adherence. Why challenge yourself when your cravings and propensity for weight gain are higher than at any other time? Wait until during or after your period, when cravings ebb. If you establish good habits in the first part of your cycle, you can maintain the diet when urges for sweet carbohydrates and fatty foods return in the second half.

Speaking of yearnings—there is now scientific evidence that

women have particularly strong cravings for chocolate (as if anyone needed proof!). A review by researchers at the University of Copenhagen showed that women crave chocolate much more than men, particularly in the luteal phase of their cycle, and that they prefer it to other types of food. The craving did not appear to be satiated by anything else. If they completely resist the desire to eat a certain food, like chocolate, many women are likely to keep snacking, taking in more calories in the process. Thus, giving in to cravings in a controlled way can prevent overeating other foods to try to satisfy the urge. If chocolate is something you need, keep on hand a small stock of the dark kind, which contains the healthier monounsaturated oleic acid, and indulge in a limited way.

Dieting doesn't have to be all or nothing, and, in fact, it shouldn't be. Such dichotomous thinking is also a weakness of women—women who go off of their diet have more of a tendency than men to believe they have failed and should stop trying. The psychology of forgiveness, and the will to get right back on track, can save weeks' worth of effort for women dieters (see chapter 8).

Habits of Successful Dieters

Dieters can learn a lot from others who have effectively controlled their weight. Luckily, there are several good databases of information. Rena Wing and James Hill started the National Weight Control Registry (NWCR) in 1994 to study why some people have long-term success with weight loss while others do not. They've tracked over four thousand dieters who've lost thirty pounds or more and kept it off for at least one year. The Diabetes Prevention Program (DPP) and Look AHEAD (Action for Health in Diabetes) are also registries that track behavioral treatment programs. The information they collect tells us that successful dieters have many things in common:

1. They often have an emotional trigger or life event that provokes them to start and stay on a diet.
2. Most don't go off their diets, even on holidays and weekends, and exhibit a high level of self-control as measured in cognitive restraint tests.

3. They use self-monitoring tools to maintain a detailed log of their weight, calories, and activities.

4. Those who are able to maintain weight loss for two years are more likely to maintain the loss.

5. They exercise the equivalent of one hour per day of moderate-intensity exercise such as brisk walking, overall expending 2,500–3,000 calories per week in exercise. (Alternatively, vigorous exercise for 35 minutes per day also maintains loss.)

One study by Wing detailed how, for 83 percent of NWCR registrants, a specific event caused them to finally take weight loss seriously. Most often it was a medical event, such as a physician telling them to lose weight or a serious heart issue of a family member. The second most common trigger was reaching an all-time high weight. The shock of being heavier than ever before inspired people to action. Similarly, seeing a picture or reflection of themselves looking obese was a powerful incentive for many successful dieters.

Once they start dieting, successful dieters don't go off the rails frequently. They do not relax the rules much on holidays or weekends, even when everyone else is celebrating. Diet diligence made them one and a half times more likely to maintain their weight loss to within five pounds compared to people who went overboard and ate a whole fruitcake at Christmas.

It is hard to stay on a diet 100 percent of the time. But when successful dieters slip, they recover and get back on the program within days, often with the help of a weight-loss coach. Dr. Michael Dansinger coaches his patients back onto their diet by using a carefully measured strictness scale that allows them to go off the plan to some extent. He says, "I always urge people to get as close to 90 percent on a diet plan as they can. If people saw that 70 percent effort gave 70 percent of results, most people would take that deal. But unfortunately, 70 percent effort only gives about 50 percent results. Most people do well above 80 percent to get satisfying results. Why put in 75 percent effort if you're not going to get much payoff? It's kind of a rip off." To make sure they are staying at 80 percent compliance or better, Dansinger meets with patients weekly to measure their weight and track their progress. If they go off the diet, he gives them a pep talk and coaches them back on.

Terry, one of Dansinger's patients, says, "Over Christmas break when I gained a little bit back, Dr. Dansinger told me that I've come so far and that it's not worth it to lose all the work that I've done." There was no punishment or guilt, instead Dansinger's pep talk gave Terry encouragement and a great sense of relief. She adds, "So then I thought 'all right, I can have an ice cream bar, but I'm not going to jeopardize all the work that I've done to get here.' It stops me from going overboard with it." Accepting your mistake and returning to the plan after a transgression is imperative. Using a coach or dieting support group to help can make all the difference.

According to research of successful dieters, gaining a few pounds back after some weight loss is common. But those who are able to shed that small gain quickly and get back on track have a much better chance for long-term success.

Food Accounting 101

Self-monitoring is an excellent tool to minimize weight regain. Thomas Wadden at the University of Pennsylvania has studied the results from diabetes and obesity intervention programs. He's observed that those who lose the most weight consistently keep a record of calories and frequently weigh themselves. Dansinger agrees, "I found that food logging is so crucially important to progress that I insist on it. I train people how to log their food if they're struggling with it. I wish it wasn't the case because it's kind of a nuisance for people. But everyone who has achieved good results with me has been willing to do food logging. Everyone who's declined has been unable to get results." He suggests online apps that can be used from a smartphone, such as Lose It! and MyFitnessPal. But he says even using old-fashioned pen and paper is a good way to start.

Food logging is not only important for you to monitor your own intake, but so that others can see it too. Dansinger continues, "A food log is necessary, but the other issue is people won't keep a food log unless someone else is looking at it. You can monitor your own food log for a few months, but after a while you just stop. However, if you know that someone is going to look at it with you, that makes all the difference." Indeed, all the successful dieters I interviewed had a team of people helping with their food log and weight-loss program at the start: a physician, a nurse, a weight-loss coach, or someone to whom they felt accountable to monitor their progress and encourage them.

Practitioners who specialize in weight loss all agree on the importance of staying in close contact with their patients. Almost every program with a high success rate includes meeting with people frequently at first, usually weekly, then tapering down to monthly visits. They go over their patients' food log with them. They offer education, counseling, physical monitoring, and medical interventions when necessary. Once patients have weight loss under control, visits taper to biweekly, then monthly, then every few months, sometimes for years.

Dr. Louis Aronne directs the Center for Weight Management and Metabolic Clinical Research at Weill-Cornell Medical College and is a recognized leader in obesity treatment. He says, "It's a no brainer to prescribe a diet. But getting people to stick with it, that is hard. And so, you have a question of why does obesity happen? Well, it happens because it's really hard and people are really hungry. Losing it is like trying to hold your breath underwater. Tell someone to hold his breath underwater for ten minutes. And it's like 'Wow, look at that!' But could I do that? No, I couldn't."

Just as we don't treat diabetics by telling them to just eat less sugar, we can't undo obesity by simply telling people to eat less food. It's not that simple. Fat fights to keep its territory. People have one of the biggest battles of their lives trying to reclaim control. To beat the odds against maintaining weight loss, they need support.

Randy credits his impressive and permanent weight loss to the program run by doctors Richard Atkinson and Nikhil Dhurandhar (see chapter 6). For two years, Randy came to sessions, classes, and appointments. For the first three months he came several days per week, then reduced attendance to every one to two weeks and then to every one to two months for the remainder of the program. Patients who started regaining weight were asked to attend meetings more frequently. Randy says of the start of the program, "Every week you got a one hour and fifteen minute university lecture that covered the research on obesity. We started learning about studies in twins, why different people have different metabolism and why various studies were adapted into the program. Once I understood all of that, it was like 'Wow! I can do this!' I lived seventy-five miles from Madison and I couldn't wait to get there! Everyone was so eager to learn every week. The program went on for two years. People cried when it ended."

Once excess fat is established on our bodies, reducing it is a monumental effort—it becomes resistant to weight-loss efforts. If you've never been heavy in the past, you can eat more throughout your life and take a few pounds off with ease. However, if you are overweight or have been, which is the situation for most dieters, fat loss is by far more difficult. The key is to be patient and have realistic goals. You may not look like a supermodel, or even like you did when you were twenty, but you can get to a healthier and more content body with long-term effort. So long as you understand your fat and what you're up against.

Chapter 11

Mind over Fat

A significant component of successful weight loss is our ability to maintain will power. When hunger, cravings, and dissatisfaction constantly tug at us, they challenge our resolve. Many people who have successfully lost weight feel an extreme ongoing desire for food and eventually give in, regaining the pounds they so painstakingly lost.

Dr. Ancel Keys at the University of Minnesota performed one study that revealed the overwhelming effect hunger has. Keys started his study in 1944, as World War II was coming to an end, when Allied forces spread through Europe and discovered emaciated victims of war who had been held in prison camps, starved, overworked, and brought near death. Medical workers were eager to renourish them and bring them back to health, but at the time not much was known about how to treat starvation.

Keys, a professor of physiology, decided to investigate. He gathered a group of conscientious objectors—American draftees who refused to serve in the military because of their pacifist beliefs. In lieu of fighting, the objectors had to choose from a list of civilian public services such as soil conservation, forest maintenance, or volunteering for medical experiments. Four hundred men applied to take part in the study, though Keys selected only thirty-six, based on their strong physical and mental health.

Keys put these subjects on a diet averaging 1,570 daily calories, consisting mostly of potatoes, bread, turnips, and cabbage and a token amount of protein and fat—a carb-heavy regimen that approximated typical meals in war-torn Europe. In addition, the men were assigned physical activities that included twenty-two miles of walking per week, producing a calorie deficit. This starvation period lasted for six months, and during it the men were expected to lose a total of about 25 percent of their body weight.

What made this research so remarkable was the surprising psychological and physical reactions that prolonged hunger caused. As the starvation period progressed, the subjects became more lethargic and irritable. Said one, "We became, in a sense, more introverted, and we had less energy." Climbing stairs became an ordeal. One participant said, "I knew where all the elevators were in the buildings." Another said that on their walks they looked for driveways so they didn't have to expend energy by stepping up onto the curb. Resentment developed against anyone who was given a larger food ration. One participant described feeling hate for a young boy whizzing by on a bicycle, knowing that he was probably rushing home for supper.

The subjects became obsessed with food, and some developed complex behaviors around it. One recalls that "eating became a ritual. . . . Some people diluted their food with water to make it seem like more. Others would put each little bite and hold it in their mouth a long time to savor it. So eating took a long time." The men collected cookbooks and recipes. One subject remembers, "I don't know many other things in my life that I looked forward to being over with any more than this experiment. And it wasn't so much . . . because of the physical discomfort, but because it made food . . . the one central and only thing really in one's life. And life is pretty dull if that's the only thing. I mean, if you went to a movie, you weren't particularly interested in the love scenes, but you noticed every time they ate and what they ate."

Keys's landmark study displayed the immense power of hunger to affect our minds. Even though dieters may not be subjecting themselves to the same extreme measures as these study participants, they experience a prolonged hunger that is extremely difficult to resist for long periods of time. Now, modern research methods have provided some insight into the reasons why.

As discussed in chapter 5, Michael Rosenbaum and Joy Hirsch

at Columbia University analyzed brain activity in dieters using functional magnetic resonance imaging (fMRI), a tool that helps researchers visualize the parts of the brain that are active when subjects respond to stimuli. In their experiment, Rosenbaum and Hirsch studied dieters who had recently lost weight. They measured how their brains responded while viewing images of candy, grapes, broccoli, cell phones, and yo-yos. When pictures of food flashed by, brain segments associated with emotional response to food lit up brightly on the fMRI screen, but the parts of the brain associated with control were dim, indicating a low response. This means that after we lose weight, our brains are more responsive to food, but our ability to control food intake is weaker.

Rosenbaum explains that after weight loss, we experience a larger emotional response to food, so a dieter's urge to eat is possibly even stronger than before. At the same time, areas of the brain that participate in restraint have a diminished response. So we are hungrier, but our self-control is down. Combined with all the other ways that fat fights to survive (discussed in chapter 5), the stronger urges combined with diminished restraint create the perfect situation for weight regain. This condition can last for six years or possibly longer after weight has been lost.

Much of this effect is due to lower levels of leptin, the hormone emitted from fat that signals to our brain we are full. Dieting results in decreased fat mass, which lowers leptin levels, and thus we are driven towards food. Leptin is so powerful that when weight-reduced research subjects are given experimental injections of the protein, the strong effects of hunger fade (see chapter 5).

Your Self-Control "Muscles"

So how do we fight fat when fat is controlling our thoughts? Unless leptin replacement therapy becomes an approved treatment, self-control is one of the few remedies we have. Even if we cut carbs and eat plenty of protein to curb hunger, the urge to eat will be intense during weight loss. Luckily, research shows, there are ways to strengthen our ability to control that urge.

Doctors Mark Muraven of the Department of Psychology, State

University of New York at Albany, and Roy Baumeister at Florida State University have demonstrated that self-control can be strengthened, much like a muscle. By practicing on small challenges, then working toward more difficult ones, people can develop much stronger willpower. For example, researchers have found that those who exerted self-control to regulate their posture for two weeks improved at tasks that involved physical discomfort. Another study showed that those who practiced not cursing or using colloquialisms also improved their ability to regulate behavior. The particular action being taken is not what's important as long as it requires the person to inhibit a natural response. Muraven says, "People can practice small acts of self-control, like cutting back on sweets or trying not to swear. If successful, you can take on bigger acts, like quitting smoking or dealing with stress. So you can build that muscle and improve self-control."

There are fMRI studies that support the power of self-control for successful dieters. Dr. Rena Wing at Brown University, cofounder of the National Weight Control Registry, collaborated with a research team to study the brains of obese and normal-weight subjects as well as those of successful dieters who had dropped at least thirty pounds and kept it off for a minimum of three years. The researchers asked all groups to hold lemon lollipops in their mouths during fMRI scanning and evaluated their brain activity. Though the part of the brain involved in reward lit up for all groups, it was stronger for those who lost weight (similar to Rudy Leibel's studies described in chapter 5). But something unique emerged— the parts of the brain involved in restraint also lit up brightly for successful dieters, but not so much for the obese or normal-weight. That implies that among the subjects who successfully maintained weight loss, the part of the brain that controls behavior took over the organ's emotional center. These were the people who could clearly decide whether or not to eat in the face of temptation.

Studies of the National Weight Control Registry also show that members who were successful at long-term weight loss reinforced self-control regularly by implementing strict diet plans, diligent exercise routines, counting calories, and weighing themselves frequently, without taking breaks on holidays and weekends.

This research suggests the usefulness of prediet exercises to first build your self-control "muscles" before addressing bigger challenges such as sustained weight loss regimen. One could start with noneating-related tasks by, for example, committing to make the bed within thirty minutes after waking up, and then take on another task, such as cutting out a type of food, like cookies or chips. Having a successive number of small wins gives a feeling of confidence, which builds over time. Inching your way toward controlling food rather than adopting an all-or-nothing approach builds a foundation for future success.

There are further benefits to strengthening the self-control muscle. Dieting and feeling hunger produces stress, but small acts of self-control alleviate it. Muraven says, "Some of our unpublished research shows that building strength also helps with stress overall. When we had people try cutting back on swearing, they managed stress better, too. The physiological response to stress was smaller, their negative moods were lessened, and they had reported coping better than people doing other things."

Dr. Katherine Milkman studies the science of self-control and its impact on decision making at the University of Pennsylvania. A youthful professor who radiates enthusiasm, she has been recognized as an expert in her field. Milkman's work operates on the premise that we each have two selves—one that is controlled, thoughtful, and focused on the future, which she calls the "should" self, and a separate one in competition, the impulsive "want" self. It's not unlike the angel whispering in one ear, and the devil whispering in the other. Milkman says, "They exist in a state of conflict. So when there's a choice between the things we want to do and the things that we know we should do, like a decision whether to save or spend, there's tension. These things exist in a balance, but there are a lot of different factors that can tip the scales."

One thing that can shift the decision between "want" and "should" is timing. Milkman says, "When we make a choice for the present, people tend to choose what they want. When we make a decision about tomorrow, we choose what we should do. Say, when we come home after a day's work and we want comfort food and a beer, but tomorrow, we plan to exercise." The problem is that tomorrow finally becomes today, and if we constantly choose the "want" self, it weakens the "should" self.

Doctors Samuel McClure of Arizona State University and Jonathan Cohen of Princeton University were able to actually visualize the "should" and "want" parts of the human brain. Using fMRI, they saw that the limbic and paralimbic systems are activated when test subjects considered near-term reward (the "want" self), the same areas of the brain that are commonly implicated in impulsive behavior and drug addiction. On the other hand, the lateral prefrontal regions were activated when the subjects made long-term decisions (the "should" self), linking these areas to delayed gratification. Repeatedly exercising a "should" activity strengthens the part of the brain responsible for self-control. This finding supports Muraven's conclusion that practicing small acts of willpower increased subjects' ability to take on bigger tasks involving self-control.

Temptation Bundling

One approach to fighting wayward urges involves "temptation bundling," in which subjects couple a "want" activity with a "should." In one experiment, Milkman divided participants into three groups. The *full* group was allowed to listen to audio novels of their choice only at the gym; after their workouts, the novels were locked away. The *intermediate* group was allowed to keep the audio novels but was encouraged to listen only at the gym. The third, *unrestricted* group was not limited in any way and could listen to novels whenever they chose. At the start of a nine-week intervention, the full group visited the gym 51 percent more often than the unrestricted group. The intermediates visited the gym 29 percent more than the unrestricteds. Meaning: pairing a "want" activity (listening to a juicy audiobook) with a "should" one (going to the gym) was a strong incentive to exercise. The method was so valuable that when the experiment was done, 61 percent of the participants opted to pay the gym to restrict access to their audiobooks. The effect fades over several months, though, so people have to switch the "want" activity to stay engaged.

Even so, these results open up multitudes of possibilities. If we pair an unappealing chore with something we like to do, we increase the odds that we'll perform the challenging task. For example, you could buy yourself an item of clothing every week you lose some weight. This will force you to assess your body and give you a reward for being disciplined. This is temptation bundling, but it's also giving yourself a break from a constant stream of "should" activities. It recharges your brain and makes you stronger for the next time a little self-control is required (see below, "Don't Overdo It").

Another method of improving self-control is the use of pre-commitment devices, which allow you to lock in good behavior tomorrow based on your good intentions today. An example of this is a website called stickK.com that helps people create commitment contracts. On the site you create a contract with yourself in which you set a goal—for example, losing ten pounds by a specified date. You deposit money into an account and then you select a trainer or coach to referee and confirm whether or not you achieved your goal. If you don't hit your target, you lose that money. The process ensures that once tomorrow becomes today, you'll feel a strong pinch if you break the contract. For example, you can commit to giving $500 to charity if you don't achieve your goal by the specified date. Or choose an anticharity, meaning if you fail you must give money to an organization you *don't* want to help, such as the opposing political party, which is an extra incentive not to fail. Using precommitment devices is a way of forcing your future self to do what your present self thinks it should.

Fresh Starts

In Chapter 10 we discussed triggers that incite people to lose weight, such as a medical diagnosis, unexpectedly catching a glimpse of one's reflection, or hitting an all-time high number on the scale. Special dates can serve as triggers too, building on the idea of New Year's resolutions. The psychological basis of fresh starts is that all our past failures are behind us and we have a clean slate because of the new year. "That was the old me," we say. "I fell off of the wagon, I failed to diet or quit smoking, but the new me has this under control." We categorize older failures into a separate mental account. This is surprisingly effective when it comes to making lifestyle changes.

It's not just the start of a new year that can enable this change—there are many other times when we feel as though a new cycle is beginning. Milkman says, "In the beginning of a new month, or new week, following birthdays, and following holidays people seek segregation from their past selves, their past failures, and that seems to be leading to an increase in goal pursuits. So people are more likely to search for the diet following those different temporal landmarks. They're more likely to go to the gym. They're also more likely to create precommitment contracts."

There is evidence that this new-start phenomenon can be turned on and off just by simple framing. Milkman explains, "When we describe March 20th as the first day of spring as opposed to just mentioning it's the third Thursday in March, we see more people getting excited about receiving a reminder on that date to pursue goals they want to pursue. That feels like a fresh start. So people can try to create fresh starts and take advantage of that thinking where they feel separated from the past failures and feel strong enough to tackle new goals, even if they've gone off the rails in the past."

Don't Overdo It

One note of caution, however. Like any muscle, overuse of willpower causes fatigue. With too much exertion, the self-control part of our brain gets worn out. Milkman's research showed that caregivers in hospitals dramatically decrease the rate at which they perform "should" activities as an exhausting day progresses. For example, workers become less likely to wash their hands—a "should"—late in the day. And the more intense the workday is, the more pronounced the decline.

In another study, Muraven and his team assembled study subjects who had been asked to skip a meal. He then divided the group into two, and made freshly baked chocolate chip cookies available to one group, and radishes available to the other. He asked both groups to abstain from eating the other group's food. Naturally, the cookies were a hit with these hungry participants. But the group that had to consistently exercise willpower by avoiding cookies and limiting themselves to radishes had less persistence in solving puzzles afterward. They showed more frustration and gave up more easily than those allowed to freely eat the cookies. The constant exertion of self-control wore them out.

Fortunately, this fatigue can be reversed. Research by Dr. Dianne Tice at Florida State University showed that enjoying a pleasant activity can restore the willpower depleted by too much self-denial. Her research team asked study participants to maintain a strong grip on a hand exerciser for as long as possible. At break time the subjects were assigned to watch either a sad or humorous movie clip before continuing the exercise. The group that watched the humorous movie was able to continue the hand-gripping exercise for longer than those who watched the sad movie. And Milkman and team found that health-care workers continue to wash their hands regularly if they take longer breaks between shifts. The key to getting back is taking a rest, or finally indulging in a want activity.

Be careful about *how* you give in to the activity you are trying to control, though. Consider the "abstinence violation effect," which shows that for many people, one slipup is followed by additional slips, which justify allowing oneself even more. Muraven says, "It's so much easier to maintain a bright line to say 'never again,' otherwise people can fall down a slippery slope. People tend to say, if I have this once, what's the difference between one and two? Or I had one yesterday why not have one today too and then it just goes on from there." So, if you stumble once, pick yourself up quickly and try not to do it again. And, when you do indulge in a "want" activity, pick one that doesn't involve the food with the potential to throw you off course.

Uncertainty and Stress

The *New York Times* reported that during the time of uncertainty caused by the 2008–2009 economic crisis, sales of candy soared as other consumer purchases declined. Some stores had a hard time keeping sweets in stock; customers said that even though they had less money, they kept funds aside for candy. Profits of candy corporations soared by double digits, even though other companies were reporting big declines. Sales of candy also soared during the Great Depression, amid constant negative headlines about the market and portfolios at a fraction of their previous value. With an uncertain future, people were in a state of anxiety, which took a toll on willpower.

This isn't just a convenient anecdote. Studies have shown that a lack of control in our environment chips away at our willpower and ability to manage stress. A 1969 study by D. C. Glass separated subjects into two groups: one was forced to listen to unpredictable noise, while the other had the power to turn off the racket. Those with no control had less ability to apply themselves to solving puzzles later. Another experiment, by Dr. Drury Sherrod at Kirkland College, showed that people in a crowded room were better able to manage stress if they believed they had an option to leave compared to those who did not.

If we feel uncertainty in our daily lives, whether over a medical test, job offer, or family situation, the lingering doubt depletes our willpower. Starting a weight-management plan during such a time of uncertainty makes it more difficult to persevere. If it is possible to ease the stress in your life before starting a serious attempt to change your lifestyle, do so. Successful weight management requires the ability to take challenges in stride and maintain your diet and exercise plan.

The good news is that as you practice the "should" behaviors, they will turn into habits that require less effort to execute. Doctors Gary Charness and Uri Gneezy of the University of California ran an experiment in which they paid one group of people to exercise eight times in a month and another group to exercise just once during the same period. The next month they didn't pay anybody. The group that exercised eight times per month continued to go to the gym more often after the experiment than they had before, even though they were no longer being paid. This supports the idea that if you repeat the behavior that you want to incorporate, it will eventually become a habit. You can use this psychology to reduce overeating and adopt other healthy behaviors, even in the presence of everyday stress.

Have Meaningful Goals

Not everyone has to be a Swedish bikini model or a body builder with six-pack abs. Age, dieting history, hormones, genetics, even microbes will cause individual challenges for managing fat. What matters is that you bring your fat to a healthy level, not that you meet someone else's standard. You don't have to accept the media's war on fat and the giant industry it fuels. There is a lot of money in making people feel they have to be lean and perfect, and then selling them items that don't necessarily help in the process. Set your goals and diet plan in a way that makes sense for you.

Those who tend to go the distance on diet plans are those who are personally invested in the outcome. Muraven comments, "Research shows that for people who feel like they are doing the exercise or losing weight for personal reasons, reasons that feel important for them, it's going to be a lot easier to lose the weight. They are more successful than people who are doing it for more external reasons. So if you are losing weight because your spouse nagged you into dieting, or the doctor did, or you're going to gain the approval of your boss, you'll be less likely to succeed than if you are doing it because it matters to you." Trainer Sherry Winslow says she has more success with people who are trying to lose weight if they are personally invested: "The ones who stay with it are those who have a motivation like 'I don't want to die' or 'I want to see my kids grow up.'"

Finally, remember that your fat is part of your personal history. It's a chapter of your life story. So the effort to lose weight and maintain that loss will be harder for those of us who initially gained a significant amount of fat. We have to eat less and exercise more than our peers who have never been overweight.

For those who have a history of being overweight, however, there is some good news. Weight loss for successful dieters gets easier over time. According to an analysis of the NWCR, those who are able to keep weight off for two years, through persistence, willpower, and good habits, are able to keep it off even longer because these changes become hard-wired. Success is truly mind over fat.

Chapter 12

Fat Control II: How
I Do It

I set out on this journey to understand fat for a simple reason: I couldn't figure out why my body was so good at holding on to it. I had seen fat be stubborn, resistant, obstructionist, and elusive all at the same time. My observations led me on a scientific path to understand what fat truly is and why it behaves so differently depending on the person.

I studied the research, interviewed dozens of leading scientists, and talked to patients who struggle with it. And soon I felt armed and ready to better analyze my own situation and change it. So what were the factors that made it so easy for me to gain weight and such torture to lose?

I believe genetics was a major contributor to my weight. My mother wrestled with weight her whole life even though she put up a remarkable fight to keep it under control. She was never obese but, like me, she had about twenty to thirty pounds more than she really wanted in middle age. I remember weeks at a time when she barely ate—just a breakfast of two eggs, two pieces of toast, and a cup of tea, then nothing more than another cup of tea at dinnertime. It was her own version of intermittent fasting and balancing protein and carbs. It worked—to a point. She never became obese, and she could occasionally lose some of her softness. However, she was seldom thin, and could never really join the "eating world," as successful dieter Randy calls it. I remember feeling sorry for my mother as she cooked big dinners for us but refused to take a plate for herself.

Little did I know as a child that I had inherited her burden. My body and face closely resembled hers, and not surprisingly I also got her metabolism and propensity for fat.

My ancestry was weighing in as well. My family heritage is eastern Indian. And do you think my ancestors experienced adverse conditions? Why, yes. India has suffered numerous famines that have been recorded since the eleventh century. It would not surprise me if I had a thrifty genotype similar to the American Pima Indians that was helping me pack on weight. And wasn't SMAM-1, a virus that may lead to obesity, first identified in India? It is unknown whether this virus is transmissible between humans, but it hasn't been ruled out either.

I learned that bacterial flora is also shared within families. Different cultures have different gut microbes, and they can be transmitted by mother to infant. These bacteria evolve to extract nutrients from indigenous foods and allow humans to thrive in many different circumstances. So maybe my Indian lineage, with a history of adverse conditions, bestowed on me microbes that are very effective at taking every last nutrient out of my food and storing it as fat. Let's just say that I don't have a body that diverts very much to waste. What comes in tends to stay in.

So, my genetics and heritage weren't helping me stay thin. And my two X chromosomes weren't making it any easier either. I will never ever be able to eat like my Irish-Italian husband, who can wolf down thousands of calories per day and stay as thin as he was in college. So there won't be any sharing of midnight snacks before we go off to bed. When it comes to eating, you're on your own, dear.

How I treated my fat in the past also matters, it turns out. I have a history of yo-yo dieting. I went on my first diet at age twelve, and through my twenties was always losing ten pounds and gaining it back. What did this do to my fat? Constant attack made it stronger, more resilient, more skillful. As Rudy Leibel, Mike Rosenbaum, and Joseph Proietto reported, once we have fat and try to lose it, the body uses multiple mechanisms to restore it. My previous weight losses caused my metabolism to be even slower than it would have been otherwise. My muscles had become more efficient and burned fewer calories. I was always hungry. Just like the fMRI images showing that people who lose weight are more responsive to food, thoughts of eating were never too far from my mind.

Hormones were factoring in as well. My body is very sensitive to sugar. Just one small portion of dessert and I could gain a pound in a day. Insulin does its job well and puts these calories into my fat. This is a benefit in that my blood work always looks pretty good at my yearly checkup—triglycerides are mostly under control—but my jeans have a tendency to get snug. I have never been able to casually eat sugary yogurts, ice cream, or cereals the way my friends could, and stay thin. As Michael Jensen says, this ability to pack fat may have helped my blood stay clean, but it hindered my ability to lose weight.

In my forties, my fat burning hormones were slowing down. My levels of growth hormone, testosterone, and estrogen were decreasing, lowering my metabolism and lean mass, and making fat loss more difficult. That ten-pound gain or loss was a thing of the past—now I had almost thirty pounds that didn't want to move.

So I had genes, gender, age, hormones, yo-yo dieting, and possibly microbes against me. All these factors were coming together to help fat accumulate on my body and more easily resist my attempts to lose it. Apparently, I had very smart fat that knew how to survive in times of adversity. No wonder I had to eat much less than any personal trainer would ever advise to lose just a few pounds. I was on the extreme end of the bell curve, with folks who have to eat drastically less than average to be thin.

After my research, I also knew what I didn't have. I didn't have a significant gene mutation that made me obese, like the *ob* mutation or any other. If I had fat-friendly gene mutations, such as in FTO (see chapter 7), weight control would be much more challenging. I also didn't have deficiencies in my hormone levels, something I had considered when I started this research. Other than typical hormone and metabolism declines due to age, I had no serious health abnormalities. I was normal, just fat-challenged.

Well, I'm much smarter now where fat is concerned. I know a lot about it after all the research. So what do I do?

Fight. It is now my soul versus fat. Nature may have given me a body that loves fat, but it also gave me a will of steel. I've always been a determined person, and that isn't going to change. If my body was clever at putting on fat, then I would be more clever about losing it. If my fat was determined to stay, then I would be more determined to make it leave. It was mind over fat. And once my motivation was there, fat could not win.

It's not that I didn't learn to love my fat. I did. In fact, I realized just how much torment I had been putting it through all this time. I had overeaten, lost weight, then ate too much again, and my fat sat there silently, bravely absorbing it all. My fat had protected me as a baby, kick-started my puberty, fueled my reproductive system, then kindly dissolved itself when I nursed my kids, and now was sticking with me, to be used as a soft cushion in times of need.

But as much as I appreciate my fat, I also know it is not healthy for it to continue expanding as I grow older. Part of loving is having the strength to say "no," just as you would to a spoiled child. I love you, fat, but it is better for both of us if you don't stay. At least not in your current state.

So, now . . . fat and I fight. We fight, and we negotiate and we vie for the upper hand. It's not unlike a divorce with mixed emotions. But fat had all the advantages in our early battles. What is different now? I am aware of every trick fat plays. Armed with this knowledge, I persist. My genes have given fat the advantage? My hormones are slowing down? My metabolism is lower? Fine. I'll eat less. Way, *way* less.

I start with intermittent fasting. If my genes are accustomed to famine and starvation, then let them have it. I eat a small breakfast of about 200 calories at 8 a.m., and lunch of about 500 calories, and a snack at 3 p.m. of 200 calories, all balanced in roughly equal portions of carbohydrate and protein, and around 20 percent fat. I keep sugars and refined carbs very low. I skip dinner, which gives me a seventeen-hour fast each day. If hunger is too difficult at night, I eat a handful of nuts, or perhaps a little slice of cheese and hot herbal tea. That's it. If I need a distraction I flick on the TV or play a game with my kids. I get up and do the same thing day after day.

This is not easy, and my kids think it's odd that I'll cook dinner for them but won't eat it. Sound familiar? This is how I felt about my mother when I was growing up. But I don't feel sorry for myself. I feel powerful. I'm showing fat a lesson. I weigh myself every day. In two weeks, three pounds are gone. I wish I could shed more, but I've learned not to expect quick losses.

I get used to my new routine and feel strong, except that after several more weeks, only those three pounds are gone, no more. I'm on a seesaw, one pound up, two down, one up again. A month goes by like this. Only four pounds gone in total. My fat wants to play tough? Fine. I add exercise.

As Dr. Michael Dansinger says (chapter 10), it is difficult to lose all the desired weight without exercise. So I start running in the morning in a fasted state. Doing so is thought to be more effective at enhancing glucose metabolism and preventing fat accumulation than exercising later in the day, after eating. I start with thirty minutes every other day. Now we're moving—two pounds lost in one week. I add thirty minutes of strength-building exercise three times per week in between my running days. Another pound is gone. The weight loss is slow, but I tell myself I'm adding muscle. Then I plateau for two weeks. A total of five pounds lost in seven weeks. Come on!

While this is going on, I'm hungry and obsessing about food. It's just as the study by Ancel Keys showed (see chapter 11): I notice food everywhere—TV, magazines, anyone eating around me. Everything looks good. Even things I would normally find repellent, like liver and onions. I fantasize about food as I go to bed. My husband has come to expect my new routine: every night before bed I talk about what I wish I could eat. It differs every day, but oddly I don't crave sweets anymore, just good hearty foods like pizza, eggs Benedict, chicken crepes, a bacon-avocado-turkey club. It's fantasy land. My fat is fighting back like never before by controlling my mind. Leptin levels fall precipitously during fasting and growth hormone is high at night, causing my hunger to spike and my mind to seek food. But I am resolute. Forget about it, fat, I'm in charge and you can't stay. Luckily, during sleep leptin levels rise and once I wake up, cravings disappear. All those urges I had the night before are gone, as if they were a dream.

To get off this plateau, I start keeping a meticulous diet log on a spreadsheet. I count every calorie. No more than 1,000 calories per day will go into me. This is NIDDK's definition of a low-calorie diet, and is one step up from the *very* low calorie diet of no more than 800 calories. Such restricted calories are an extreme measure that not many people have to resort to, but my fat is particularly stubborn.

Since I weigh myself every day, I now start looking for trends to see how my eating correlates with the numbers on the scale. I noticed that some carbs affect me more than others. Pizza is a disaster. Even though I'll only eat it at lunch and then skip dinner, I gain a pound any time I have a slice. So now my favorite food is on the blacklist. White bread causes easy weight gain, but not whole wheat. Rice is fine in small amounts. Cookies are another bomb. I have a single 3 p.m. cookie during that time of the month (I'm a female with a sweet tooth, what do you expect?) and what happens? I gain a pound and a half. Can you believe it? Some of this is probably water, but not all. So now, cookies are off the list, even one a month. Oddly, I can eat small bits of chocolate and nothing happens. Vanilla lattes and hot chocolates don't seem to hurt me much either. Great, a new way to satiate my sweet tooth when needed. I can live with that.

Oh, and by the way—none of what I'm doing is supposed to work according to the popular thinking on diets. How many times have you heard that eating speeds up metabolism, and you need to eat enough calories to lose weight? It is a common theme of weight loss coaches and one heard often on *The Biggest Loser*. When I tried this approach at the urging of a personal trainer, I gained weight. In fact, despite two hours of exercise a day on the plans, I couldn't eat more than 1,200 calories if I wanted to lose fat.

Yet I was finding that fasting—partial starvation—worked. Fat would lose ground. And how much have we been warned against sugars and carbs? Yet I found that in moderate amounts, I could eat them in some forms and still lose weight. As Eran Segal's research shows (see chapter 10), response to food is very individual.

Now, I'm studying my diet log and figuring out exactly which foods make me lose weight. Just as microbiome research shows, salads are great and speed up weight loss. The stringy fiber in leafy greens is tough to digest, even for bacteria. Spinach and kale are giving my microbiome a run for its money. My gut bacteria are probably tilting more towards a distribution associated with leanness (see chapter 6). As I steer clear of high-calorie foods and go for raw vegetables, my microbiome extracts fewer calories from my food, and sends more out the door as waste. Hooray!

There is one problem, though. I can't seem to stay satiated after just a salad, even when I add protein and fats to it. I find myself constantly thinking about food, rummaging for what else I might eat. Then I learn a new trick. I add some postsalad carbs, such as a wholewheat dinner roll or a few gummy bears. Voilà! The hunger is gone, and I think I know why: there is research showing that insulin has a suppressive effect on food intake. My hypothesis is that these gummy bears are provoking just enough insulin to produce satiation (which explains why I always felt hungry on extremely low-carb diets). My new trick works. I stop seeking food within minutes of eating these precious carbs and get back to work.

I continue to lose weight, but slowly. After five weeks, I've shed another hard-won four pounds. Even though I'm exercising, intermittently fasting, limiting calories to 1,000 or less, reducing carbs, and eating healthy, I still lose only a pound a week if I'm lucky. My friends who diet by having just a light dinner tell me they can lose three to four pounds a week. But not me. I'm not one to be sorry for myself, though. It just strengthens my resolve to win.

At week 13, I plateau again. I exercise and barely eat, yet I've only lost ten pounds in two months. I extend my running time to forty minutes and add high-intensity interval training, or HIIT (see chapter 10). I do twenty seconds of high-intensity exercise, then ten seconds of low-intensity, for eight cycles in four minutes and work it into my every other day forty-minute run. The weight is moving again—two more pounds in one week. I win.

All is good. Another month, five more pounds gone for a total of fifteen, but now the holidays are coming. There will undoubtedly be family and company meals to get through. I eat Thanksgiving dinner. And then leftover Thanksgiving dinner the next day.

Pecan pie two days in a row. Oh, no. I'm risking the slippery slope of dichotomous thinking, the common pitfall where dieters believe they are either completely succeeding or failing, with nothing in between. This type of thinking leads to successive failures (see chapters 8 and 10). But I am aware of this, and force myself back on track, literally. I run for fifty minutes on Saturday and get back to intermittent fasting by the Sunday after Thanksgiving. It works, but Christmas is just around the corner.

The holidays are one long plateau. There are just too many beautiful cookies around, and too much delicious food that only comes once a year. I can't help it, I indulge here and there. Remarkably, I don't gain an ounce. And this is where I learn the upside of the set point theory—just as your body will do everything it can to not lose weight, it also doesn't want to gain weight. It will just try to stay at a set point. I'm starting to like fat's tricks now.

Once January comes, I go back at it in earnest: intermittent fasting (not eating after 3 p.m.), thirty- to forty-five-minute runs every other day that work in HIIT, and I do weightlifting on alternate days to build muscle and spur growth hormone. My diet consists of a piece of bread and some protein for breakfast, or, if I am in a hurry, an energy bar. A salad with chicken and wholewheat roll for lunch, and then a little soup or my leftover salad from lunch for the 3 p.m. snack. And that's it for the day. I'm sticking to the plan: 1,000 calories or under.

The weight eventually drops again, but more slowly. I notice my resolve is now weaker. I seem to want to give in more after the holidays. The slippery slope beckons. I stay with my rules, though, forgive my mild transgressions, and get back on the plan after every stumble. But my fat has gotten smarter over the holidays. I didn't think I was really yo-yo dieting, but apparently my fickle behavior has factored in and fat is using my weaknesses to hold its ground. My body is not responding to exercise as well it used to, nor to intermittent fasting. My metabolism has likely been lowered even further, and my muscles have become even more efficient during exercise. Rats! It is a punishment for indulging.

On top of everything, I suffer a running injury—a groin pull just to remind me that I am no longer in my twenties. Thanks, body.

Now it hurts just to walk. But I don't relent. I switch to the elliptical machine and keep up my aerobics with HIIT. I stay at the same weight for all of January and half of February. I'm down, but not out. I stay the course.

Finally, third week of February, two pounds gone. The scale is moving again. But I'm now losing only two pounds a month. My fat is really fighting hard. I look pretty good, a total of seventeen pounds gone. Should I just stop? No. I want the last ten. I up the ante again and remove more carbs. Insulin, thank you for being efficient and keeping my blood clean of triglycerides and floating nutrients, but I now need you to stop depositing every spare calorie into my fat. There will be no insulin-provoking foods for a while, except for that tightly rationed dose of carbs after my salad. No more occasional sandwiches instead of salads at lunch, no more sneaking a bite of a muffin or cookie. It's over. I increase the fasting window to nineteen hours by eating only between 10 a.m. and 3 p.m., and stay diligent with my exercise for one last thrust.

One benefit—with all this exercise, I feel as though my hormones are coming back. I have more energy, I'm more upbeat, my libido is higher than it has been for years. It must be the testosterone. I seem to be less tired after exercise than in the past. My recovery time is faster. I'm guessing this is growth hormone, too. I have better muscle definition and greater strength. But alas, this regimen is time-consuming, and I think about food too often.

My fat starts to give in again, slooowly. I can lose another half pound a week, if I stick to my plan.

When I tell people about my diet, most of them think I'm crazy. No wonder my body can't lose weight, they tell me, it's in starvation mode, which is causing my body to use fewer calories. Or, they say, even the tiny amount of carbs I eat is still too much. Or, and this one I love, they tell me I'm lying. No one can *possibly* eat so little and not be skinny. I've heard it all and don't need to be judged by self-proclaimed experts anymore. I've tried every which way people have advised me to lose weight, and none of it has worked. Now, I'm doing it my way.

And by the way, if you think this diet plan is crazy, take a look at what some models and actresses do to stay thin—those who are held up as examples of what we should look like.

Models Natalia Vodianova and Kira Dikhtyar and actors Patricia Heaton, Marcia Cross, and Matthew McConaughey are just a handful of the people who have talked at length about the extreme measures that models and actors take to look thin. Some starve for days on end, eat cotton balls dipped in juice to kill hunger (this will certainly challenge the microbiome!), and use laxatives and colonic cleansers to lose weight. Some don't eat more than 500 calories per day. In an interview when she was fifty-one, Patricia Heaton said she fasts to lose weight and drinks only three bottles of water each day. Much worse, some models take drugs, both legal and illegal, to stay thin. And these are the diets behind the figures we idolize? No thank you. In comparison, my 1,000 calories per day and partial fast looks like outrageous gluttony. I'll stay with my plan.

I endure another trying three months of hunger, exercise, and precise time management that would make a German engineer proud. And guess what? By summer, the last ten pounds are finally gone. I win. Fat has conceded territory on my body. My skinny jeans are back on. It took a battle of wills but it is done. And you know what? My fat doesn't seem unhappy. As time passes, it is no longer making me hungry all the time. I don't gain it back so easily even when I transgress now and then. My body has changed. It seems to anticipate my nightly fast. I can feel it get ready right around 5 p.m.—I feel a certain calm as I head into the foodless hours. Now my body doesn't even want a normal meal at night. I feel uncomfortably full after a birthday outing or business dinner. I do still crave certain foods right before bed, but the urges are less intense. I've come to associate hunger pangs with an earnest day of dieting.

When I started this plan, I hated exercising. It was a chore. Now my body gets antsy if I skip a few days. It wants to get back on the treadmill. It's as though my body has adjusted to a new reality. Fat has grown comfortable with its diminished role in my body and my weight has moved to a new set point.

But I am not deceived by my hard-won success. I know my fat is waiting patiently, ready to come back if I slip too many times. I can't let up on my diet and exercise if I want to keep my weight down. Like the subjects tracked in the NWCR database, I'll continue to maintain a log of what I eat, because it makes me more conscious of my intake. I'll probably increase my eating window back to seven hours, but I'll continue to eat less and exercise more than most middle-aged people do. It's what my body demands. But I am not bitter. Fat and I are at peace, aware and respectful of each other's power.

For anyone trying to manage fat, I wish you not only the required strength and determination, but also the necessary open-mindedness to understand your fat. There are multifaceted reasons why you may be thinner or heavier than your peers, and gluttony, the usual suspect, is just one of them. Having read this book, you know that genetics, bacteria, gender, age, heritage, hormones, and dieting history are factors that work for you or against you when you attempt to change your weight. If excess fat has resided on your body for over a year, manipulating internal resources, then losing it will be an all-consuming endeavor.

Fear not, it can be done. I, and other successful dieters, provide a living testament of the enormous power of personal drive—mind over fat. Enlist your passion, competitive spirit, anger, vengeance, whatever feelings your situation evokes, to take on your fat. Adipose is a major trickster, and you will need all of your mental tools to win.

But somewhere in your battle, don't forget to love and respect your fat. Fat may have grown a little self-important while we accumulated large amounts of it, but it still plays a vital role in our bodies. Once you get it to a healthy level, and in the right locations, fat will return to serving you well and keeping you healthy.

Chapter 13

The Future of Fat

So much knowledge has been gained since Theodore Gobley, David Rittenberg, Rudolph Schoenheimer, and others first characterized the fat molecule at the turn of the twentieth century. And with such remarkable leaps in insight, who knows what else we may discover? Ongoing studies are already telling us that fat has capabilities well beyond our expectations.

It's recently been shown that adipose tissue is a storage house of stem cells—those chameleon-like cells capable of turning into nerves, muscles, bone, and fat. Nature creates stem cells to ensure that the most important tissues of our bodies will be produced when necessary, and, remarkably, fat is included in this distinguished list. Not only can it be created from stem cells, but it can also store them.

Finding stem cells in fat surprised scientists. It had long been known that embryos contain stem cells that create tissues in the developing body. Less potent stem cells were also known to exist in adult bone marrow. Then, in 2001, scientist Patricia Zuk and her team at UCLA took a close look at fat sucked out of buttocks, hips, and stomachs of patients undergoing liposuction and discovered what came to be called adipose derived stem cells (ASCs). Just a half pound of fat could yield 50 to 100 million stem cells. "Most people think that fat is useless. But we found that it carries these very important cells that give rise to many different tissues." Zuk continues, "No one in the world had published this before and there was a remarkable amount of interest from the press. People were amazed that fat could be used as a therapy."

It makes sense for ASCs to be in fat—it enables them to be widely distributed in the body to replace important tissues as needed. And once harvested, ASCs have potential for regenerating soft tissue and growing bone, muscle, and cartilage on demand. Fat, that much maligned organ, could end up being critical for treating injuries and burns, or even cancer patients needing replacement tissues.

Since Zuk's discovery in 2001, progress has been made towards realizing the potential of these cells. In 2004, Dr. Stefan Lendeckel used ASCs to fix the skull of a seven-year-old girl with severe head injury. Years later, Dr. Eckhard Alt of MD Anderson in Texas tested ASCs in the hearts of pigs that had suffered heart attacks. After only eight weeks, pigs that received ASCs had better heart function compared to those that didn't. ASCs have repeatedly shown potential to hasten the healing of skin wounds. For example, researchers in China added ASCs to the wounds of diabetic and normal rats, and found that the cells significantly accelerated healing by secreting numerous growth factors that help regenerate skin.

Texas governor Rick Perry made the news in 2011 when he used ASC treatment to alleviate pain in his back. He had ASCs taken from his own fat, grown in a laboratory, and then injected back into his body during surgery. His chief of staff reported that Perry was very pleased with the results and rapid recovery. The procedure, however, was not FDA-approved, which made it controversial.

Not surprisingly, ASCs are now being used for cosmetic procedures too. Dr. Sharon McQuillan, a cosmetic surgeon and founder of the Ageless Aesthetic Institute in Florida, told the *Miami Herald*, "We can put a youthful blanket of fat over the muscles in the face so you don't see the crows' feet anymore." At the age of sixty-three Donna Arnold had cosmetic work done by McQuillan, who liposuctioned fat from Arnold's waist and injected it into a number of sites on her face. Arnold said, "The wrinkles are gone. I feel healthier and better. I'm back to exercising every day and taking better care of myself."

The procedure is not just transferring fat, as in fat grafts, which can diminish with time. ASCs are thought to be more malleable and to secrete many needed growth factors to help keep the effects in place for much longer.

Fat has even more to offer than stem cells. Brown fat could end up being a treatment to reduce unhealthy fat. Dr. Kristin Stanford of the Joslin Diabetes Center in Boston transplanted brown fat from one mouse into the abdominal cavity of a group of overweight mice. She compared the results of this transplantation to a control group of overweight mice that received abdominal transplants of white fat instead. Stanford found that after twelve weeks, the mice that got brown fat responded to insulin better, weighed less, and burned more calories than the control group, even though both groups of mice were eating the same diet. Stanford says, "This study provides further evidence that BAT [brown adipose tissue] is a very important metabolic organ and a potential treatment for obesity-related diseases such as diabetes, metabolic syndrome, and insulin resistance."

Now the potential of stem cells and brown fat are even coming together. Dr. Paul Lee, an endocrinologist at the Garvan Institute in Sydney, has been studying the ability of fat-derived stem cells to turn into brown fat. Lee and his team have been able to grow a person's brown fat outside the body. The possibility of then reinjecting brown fat could be a way to burn white fat. "We know almost all humans have some brown fat. Some have more, some have less, but it's there," Dr. Lee says. "If we can get the conditions right, we can potentially stimulate the growth of it in humans. Or we could harvest the human brown fat cells, grow them in a laboratory, then put them back into the body to increase the amount." It sounds far-fetched, growing brown fat to help get rid of white fat, but scientists think it's plausible.

There are ways to try to activate brown fat naturally as well. Dr. Lee has done experiments in which subjects are exposed to cold temperatures until they begin shivering. Lee noticed that levels of irisin, the protein produced by muscle, and FGF21, a protein emitted by brown fat, both rose significantly. The two proteins together have been known to turn white fat cells into brown after six days in the lab. In humans, after ten to fifteen minutes of shivering, subjects produced as much irisin as if they had done an hour of moderate exercise. Lee says, "We speculate exercise could be mimicking shivering—because there is muscle contraction during both processes, and that exercise-stimulated irisin could have evolved from shivering in the cold." Who needs tennis? A cold swim anyone?

Reducing Obesity Is a Team Event

New adipose research reinforces the idea that fat is intertwined with our brain, bones, immunity, hormones, genes, microbiome, and even our stem cells. As research continues, it is likely we will uncover even more surprising insights.

But despite all the exciting new knowledge, the treatment of overweight individuals hasn't changed much. Obesity is something people are judged for. Having too much fat is still considered irresponsible, weak, and gluttonous, and society still doesn't appreciate the challenge of reducing it. The common advice to the overweight remains simply to burn more calories than one consumes, with no consideration given to what science tells us about the various ways fat will defend itself.

Currently, physicians give overweight patients an empathetic and thoughtful talk on the dangers of obesity, followed by straightforward advice on reducing calories, and then send them on their way. But this one-time lecture will probably never lead to permanent weight loss.

Diabetes was once also treated very simply, before the medical community recognized its multidimensional nature. Until the discovery of insulin in 1922, no one could do much to treat it. Patients presented with symptoms such as high glucose in the urine, and without any adequate treatment would slowly die. Frederick Allen, a physician and researcher in the early 1900s, was the first to observe that diabetes was more than just high blood sugar: it was a metabolic disorder. He created its first treatment—a restricted-calorie diet consisting primarily of protein and fats with only the minimum amount of carbohydrates. Many patients followed the plan and stayed alive for years longer than had previously been possible.

Since then, treatment has changed dramatically. When a patient is diagnosed with diabetes, a medical team is assembled to properly manage the disease. This team may consist of the primary-care physician, an endocrinologist, a dietician, an eye doctor, a podiatrist, and a dentist to deal with all the ramifications of the disease. The patients still have responsibility to manage their condition, but they are helped by a coordinated team of experts.

We are still in the early days of treating obesity, but it is possible to imagine a day when obesity will be treated with as much seriousness and coordination as diabetes is now.

With climbing obesity rates driving health-care costs, regulatory officials are starting to think differently about fat. The Treat and Reduce Obesity Act drafted in 2013 by Congress would allow both physicians and nonphysicians to be reimbursed for behavioral therapy for obesity. Medications would also be covered under Medicare. Also in 2013, the American Medical Association recognized obesity as a disease that requires medical intervention. AMA board member Patrice Harris said, "Recognizing obesity as a disease will help change the way the medical community tackles this complex issue that affects approximately one in three Americans," again opening the door for possible reimbursement to treat the disease.

All this is good news, but even these actions do nothing to prevent obesity in the first place. It is much easier to maintain one's weight than to reduce it. Even with the new guidelines, most health-care insurance only covers medical intervention when there is a BMI of 35 or higher, a level only reached by the extremely obese. Many of the overweight would therefore have to gain more before becoming eligible for reimbursement. But by the time someone has reached this stage, it is much harder to reduce fat, which is now embedded, scheming and planning its ways to survive. Medical interventions at this point are costly and more risky, and the long term success rate less sure.

We'd all be better served by funding preventive measures. Individuals in high-risk situations, such as those with a family history of obesity, would particularly benefit from early intervention through a nutritionist or coach. It would save billions down the road. We'll wake up to that fact sooner or later.

And when we do, will that be the end of our fat obsession? Will it become just another body tissue, like muscle or bone? It's hard to imagine a world where fat isn't an object of so much fascination and revulsion. Perhaps one day fat will be respected for the benevolent and malleable organ that it is. And our efforts to manage it will be up to par with the amazing scientific research revealing its potential.

ACKNOWLEDGMENTS

The writing of this book was a monumental effort and so many people contributed at both a personal and professional level.

First and foremost, I need to acknowledge my husband, who was the first person to ever believe in this book and my ability to write it. Thanks for providing constant encouragement and taking care of everything in our lives to give me time to research and write. This book couldn't have been written without your help.

Second, I'd like to thank my agent, Richard Pine, who was the first person in the literary world to believe in this book. I still have your first e-mail with "Let's work together." Everything changed from there. You were a helpful mentor and confidant throughout the process. Appreciation also goes to everyone on the Inkwell team, including Eliza Rothstein, Lyndsey Blessing, and William Callahan.

Tom Mayer at W. W. Norton was my editor, who gave so much of himself to making this the best book it could be. I was lucky to have someone so invested. Others from W. W. Norton also contributed, including Ryan Harrington, Meredith McGinnis, Erin Lovett Sinesky, and Sarah Bolling. Bill Tonelli, Bill Phillips, David Beier, Ursheet Parikh, Laura Hamill, and the Roberts family also provided insightful editing and marketing advice. The things I've learned from working together with you all will contribute to future works.

Back to a personal note—I really do need to acknowledge my two lovely daughters, who were forever patient as their mother holed up in her office for years writing a book. I hope one day you'll both read the book and appreciate the result of your sacrifice. But for now, let's finally have some fun.

Of course, I'd like to thank all of the scientists, physicians, and patients I interviewed for sharing their stories with me. The book is much more personal, enriching, and genuine with your heartfelt stories in it. Many were also very helpful at reviewing and editing the chapters for accuracy and adding supplemental information and referrals. The world owes a debt to everyone who dedicates themselves to researching and understanding fat.

BIBLIOGRAPHY
AND
REFERENCES

Prologue—Skinny Jeans

Monica Rizzo, "Countdown to Glam!," *People*, March 3, 2008.

Valerie Bertinelli, *Losing It: And Gaining My Life Back One Pound at a Time* (New York: Atria Books, 2008).

Introduction—Our Changing Views of Fat

Barbara Walters interview with Newt Gingrich on *The 10 Most Fascinating People of 1995*, ABC.

U.S. Department of Homeland Security, *Budget-in-Brief: Fiscal Year 2014*.

The U.S. Weight Loss Market: 2014 Status Report & Forecast, Marketdata Enterprises Inc.

"Ad Buyers Bulk Up Spending as Consumers Diet," http://blog.nielsen.com/nielsen wire/consumer/ad-buyers-bulk-up-spending-as-consumers-diet, January 13, 2009.

"Adult Obesity Facts," Centers for Disease Control and Prevention, http://www.cdc .gov/obesity/data/adult.html.

"Half of Germans Are Obese and Overweight," http://www.gallup.com/poll/150359/ half-germans-obese-overweight.aspx, October 27, 2011.

"A Quarter of Germany Is Obese: Experts," *The Local*, August 7, 2013, http://www .thelocal.de/20130807/51259.

"Obesity Update: June 2014," Organisation for Economic Co-operation and Development, http://www.oecd.org/health/obesity-update.htm.

Peter Stearns, *Fat History: Bodies and Beauty in the Modern West*, 2nd ed. (New York: NYU Press, 2002).

Thomas Cation Duncan, *How To Be Plump: Or Talks On Physiological Feeding (1878)* (Whitefish, MT: Kessinger Publishing, 2010).

Elena Levy-Navarro, ed., *Historicizing Fat in Anglo-American Culture* (Columbus: The Ohio State University Press, 2010).

Lois W. Banner, *American Beauty: A Social History . . . Through Two Centuries of the American Idea, Ideal, and Image of the Beautiful Woman* (New York: Alfred A. Knopf, 1983).

Hillel Schwartz, *Never Satisfied: A Cultural History of Diets Fantasies and Fat* (New York: The Free Press, 1986).

J. L. Hargrove, "Does the History of Food Energy Units Suggest a Solution to 'Calorie Confusion'?," *Nutrition Journal* 6, no. 44 (2007): 1–11.

———, "History of the Calorie in Nutrition," *Journal of Nutrition* 136, no. 12 (December 2006): 2957–61.

Jim Painter, "How Do Food Manufacturers Calculate the Calorie Count of Packaged Foods?," *Scientific American*, July 31, 2006.

W. C. Cutting, D. A. Rytand, and M. L. Tainter, "Relationship Between Blood Cholesterol and Increased Metabolism from Dinitrophenol and Thyroid1," *Jounal of Clinical Investigation* 13, no. 4 (July 1, 1934): 547–52.

"Woman Died After Accidental Overdose of Highly Toxic Diet Pills," *The Guardian*, July 23, 2015.

Barbara Walters interview with Oprah Winfrey on *The 10 Most Fascinating People of 2014*, ABC.

1. The Foundation: Fat Does More Than You Think

Asim Kurjak and Frank A. Chervenak, eds., *Textbook of Perinatal Medicine*, 2nd ed. (Boca Raton, FL: CRC Press, 2006), p. 6.

C. M. Poissonnet, A. R. Burdi, and S. M. Garn, "The Chronology of Adipose Tissue Appearance and Distribution in the Human Fetus," *Early Human Development* 10, nos. 1–2 (September 1984): 1–11.

D. Haslam, "Obesity: A Medical History," *Obesity Reviews* 8, no. S1 (2007): 31–36.

A. Hassall, "Observations on the Development of the Fat Vesicle." *Lancet* (1849): 163–64.

G. Frühbeck, J. Gómez-Ambrosi, F. J. Muruzábal, and M. A. Burrell, "The Adipocyte: A Model for Integration of Endocrine and Metabolic Signaling in Energy Metabolism Regulation," *American Journal of Physiology—Endocrinology and Metabolism* 280, no. 6 (June 2001): E827–47, p. E828 first paragraph.

K. J. Ellis, "Human Body Composition: In Vivo Methods," *Physiological Reviews* 80, no. 2 (April 2000): 649–80.

R. Schoenheimer and D. Rittenberg, "Deuterium as an Indicator in the Study of Intermediary Metabolism: VI. Synthesis and Destruction of Fatty Acids in the Organism," *Journal of Biological Chemistry* 114 (1936): 381–96.

B. Shapiro and E. Wertheimer, "The Synthesis of Fatty Acids in Adipose Tissue in Vitro," *Journal of Biological Chemistry* 173 (1948): 725–28.

Rexford Ahima, *Metabolic Basis of Obesity* (New York: Springer Science and Business Media, 2011).

E. A. Oral et al., "Leptin-Replacement Therapy for Lipodystrophy," *New England Journal of Medicine* 346, no. 8 (February 21, 2002): 573.

"Cold Exposure Prompts Body to Convert White Fat to Calorie-burning Beige Fat," Endocrine Society, https://www.endocrine.org/news-room/press-release-

archives/2014/cold-exposure-prompts-body-to-convert-white-fat-to-calorie
-burning-beige-fat.

M. Harms and P. Seale, "Brown and Beige Fat: Development, Function and Therapeutic Potential," *Nature Medicine* 19 (October 2013): 1252–63.

R. Padidela et al., "Severe Resistance to Weight Gain, Lack of Stored Triglycerides in Adipose Tissue, Hypoglycaemia, and Increased Energy Expenditure: A Novel Disorder of Energy Homeostasis" *Hormone Research In Pædiatrics* 77, no. 4 (April 2012): 261–68.

E. Overton, "The Probable Origin and Physiological Significance of Cellular Osmotic Properties," *Vierteljahrschrift der Naturforschende Gesselschaft* (Zurich) 44, (1899): 88–135. Trans. R. B. Park, in *Biological Membrane Structure*, ed. D. Branton and R. B. Park (Boston: Little, Brown & Co., 1968), pp. 45–52.

M. Edidin, "Lipids on the Frontier: A Century of Cell-Membrane Bilayers," *Nature Reviews Molecular Cell Biology* 4, no. 5 (May 2003): 414–18.

Pierre Morell and Richard H. Quarles, "Characteristic Composition of Myelin," in *Basic Neurochemistry: Molecular, Cellular and Medical Aspects*, 6th ed., ed. G. J. Siegel, B. W. Agranoff, R. W. Albers, et al. (Philadelphia: Lippincott-Raven, 1999).

"Essential Fatty Acids: The Work of George and Mildred Burr," *The Journal of Biological Chemistry* 287, no. 42, (October 12, 2012): 35439–41.

2. Fat Can Talk

C. T. Montague et al., "Congenital Leptin Deficiency Is Associated with Severe Early-Onset Obesity in Humans," *Nature* 387, no. 6636 (June 26, 1997): 903–8.

Coleman quote taken from: D. L. Coleman, "A Historical Perspective on Leptin," *Nature Medicine* 16, no. 10 (October 2010): 1097–99.

A. M. Ingalls, M. M. Dickie, and G. D. Snell, "Obese, a New Mutation in the House Mouse," *Journal of Heredity* 41 (1950): 317–18.

D. L. Coleman, "Effects of Parabiosis of Obese with Diabetes and Normal Mice," *Diabetologia* 9 (1973): 294–98.

Y. Zhang et al., "Positional Cloning of the Mouse Obese Gene and Its Human Homologue," *Nature* 372 (1994): 425–32. (Erratum, *Nature* 374 [1995]: 479.)

J. L. Halaas et al., "Weight-Reducing Effects of the Plasma Protein Encoded by the Obese Gene," *Science* 269 (1995): 543–46.

S. Farooqi et al., "Effects of Recombinant Leptin Therapy in a Child with Congenital Leptin Deficiency," New England Journal of Medicine 341, no. 12 (September 16, 1999): 879–84.

Robert Pool, *Fat: Fighting the Obesity Epidemic* (New York: Oxford University Press, 2001).

3. Your Life Depends on Fat

Quotes from Frisch are taken from interviews as well as from: Rose E. Frisch, *Female Fertility and the Body Fat Connection* (Chicago: University of Chicago Press, 2004).

Quotes from Dr. Lawrence Vincent are taken from: Rose E. Frisch, *Female Fertility and the Body Fat Connection* (Chicago: University of Chicago Press, 2004).

R. E. Frisch and R. Revelle, "Height and Weight at Menarche and a Hypothesis of Critical Body Weights and Adolescent Events," *Science* 169, no. 3943 (July 24, 1970): 397–99.

Pam Belluck, "Rose E. Frisch, Scientist Who Linked Body Fat to Fertility, Dies at 96," *New York Times*, February 11, 2015.

R. E. Frisch and J. W. McArthur, "Menstrual Cycles: Fatness as a Determinant of Minimum Weight for Height Necessary for Their Maintenance or Onset," *Science* 185, no. 4155 (September 13, 1974): 949–51.

R. E. Frisch, G. Wyshak, and L. Vincent, "Delayed Menarche and Amenorrhea in Ballet Dancers," *New England Journal of Medicine* 303, no. 1 (July 3, 1980): 17–19.

"Ballerinas and Female Athletes Share Quadruple Health Threats," *Science Daily*, May 31, 2009, reporting on research from Medical College of Wisconsin.

Susan Donaldson James, "Female Athletes Are Too Fit to Get Pregnant," *ABC News*, Sept. 2, 2010, http://abcnews.go.com/Health/Wellness/female-athletes-compromise-fertility-intense-training-dieting/story?id=11539684.

P. K. Siiteri, "Adipose Tissue as a Source of Hormones," American Journal of Clinical Nutrition 45, no. 1 (January 1987): 277–82.

F. F. Chehab et al., "Early Onset of Reproductive Function in Normal Female Mice Treated with Leptin," *Science* 275, no. 5296 (January 1997): 88–90.

W. H. Yu et al., "Role of Leptin in Hypothalamic–Pituitary Function," *Proceedings of the National Academy of Sciences of the United States of America* 94, no. 3 (February 4, 1997): 1023–28. (Erratum, *Proceedings* 94, no. 20 [September 30, 1997]: 11108.)

A. D. Strosberg and T. Issad, "The Involvement of Leptin in Humans Revealed by Mutations in Leptin and Leptin Receptor Genes," *Trends in Pharmacological Sciences* 20, no. 6 (June 1999): 227–30.

M. Ozata, I. C. Ozdemir, and J. Licinio, "Human Leptin Deficiency Caused by a Missense Mutation: Multiple Endocrine Defects, Decreased Sympathetic Tone, and Immune System Dysfunction Indicate New Targets for Leptin Action, Greater Central Than Peripheral Resistance to the Effects of Leptin, and Spontaneous Correction of Leptin-Mediated Defects," *Journal of Clinical Endocrinology and Metabolism* 84, no. 10 (October 1999): 3686–95.

R. E. Frisch, "Body Fat, Menarche, Fitness and Fertility," *Human Reproduction* 2, no. 6 (August 1987): 521–33.

A. Strobel et al., "A Leptin Missense Mutation Associated with Hypogonadism and Morbid Obesity," *Nature Genetics* 18, no. 3 (March 1998): 213–15.

J. Licinio et al., "Phenotypic Effects of Leptin Replacement on Morbid Obesity, Diabetes Mellitus, Hypogonadism, and Behavior in Leptin-Deficient Adults," *Proceedings of the National Academy of Sciences of the United States of America* 101, no. 13 (March 30, 2004): 4531–36.

M. F. Pittinger et al., "Multilineage Potential of Adult Human Mesenchymal Stem Cells," *Science* 284, no. 5411 (April 2, 1999): 143–47.

T. Schilling et al., "Plasticity in Adipogenesis and Osteogenesis of Human Mesenchymal Stem Cells," *Molecular and Cellular Endocrinology* 271, no. 1–2 (June 15, 2007): 1–17.

M. A. Bredella et al., "Increased Bone Marrow Fat in Anorexia Nervosa," *Journal of Clinical Endocrinology and Metabolism* 94, no. 6 (June 2009): 2129–36.

W. H. Cleland, C. R. Mendelson, and E. R. Simpson, "Effects of Aging and Obesity on Aromatase Activity of Human Adipose Cells," *Journal of Clinical Endocrinology and Metabolism* 60, no. 1 (January 1985): 174–77.

A. Sayers and J. H. Tobias, "Fat Mass Exerts a Greater Effect on Cortical Bone Mass in Girls Than Boys," *Journal of Clinical Endocrinology and Metabolism* 95, no. 2 (February 2010): 699–706.

J. Shao et al., "Bone Regulates Glucose Metabolism as an Endocrine Organ Through Osteocalcin," *International Journal of Endocrinology* 2015, Article ID 967673, 9 pages, 2015.

I. R. Reid et al., "Determinants of Total Body and Regional Bone Mineral Density in Normal Postmenopausal Women—A Key Role for Fat Mass," *Journal of Clinical Endocrinology and Metabolism* 75, no. 1 (July 1992): 45–51.

D. A. Bereiter and B. Jeanrenaud, "Altered Neuroanatomical Organization in the Central Nervous System of the Genetically Obese (ob/ob) Mouse," *Brain Research* 165, no. 2 (April 13, 1979): 249–60.

R. S. Ahima, C. Bjorbaek, S. Osei, and J. S. Flier, "Regulation of Neuronal and Glial Proteins by Leptin: Implications for Brain Development," *Endocrinology* 140, no. 6 (June 1999): 2755–62.

A. Joos et al., "Voxel-Based Morphometry in Eating Disorders: Correlation of Psychopathology with Grey Matter Volume," *Psychiatry Research* 182, no. 2 (May 30, 2010): 146–51.

R. A. Whitmer et al., "Central Obesity and Increased Risk of Dementia More Than Three Decades Later," *Neurology* 71, no. 14 (September 30, 2008): 1057–64.

S. Debette et al., "Visceral Fat is Associated with Lower Brain Volume in Healthy Middle-Aged Adults," *Annals of Neurology* 68, no. 2 (August 2010): 136–44.

K. J. Anstey et al., "Body Mass Index in Midlife and Late-Life as a Risk Factor for Dementia: A Meta-Analysis of Prospective Studies," *Obesity Reviews* 12, no. 5 (May 2011): e426–37.

N. Qizilbash et al., "BMI and Risk of Dementia in Two Million People over Two Decades: A Retrospective Cohort Study," *Lancet Diabetes & Endocrinology* 3, no. 6 (June 2015): 431–36.

Quotes from Judah Folkman and Rocío Sierra-Honigmann are taken from: M. Barinaga, "Leptin Sparks Blood Vessel Growth," *Science* 281, no. 5383 (September 11, 1998): 1582.

M. R. Sierra-Honigmann et al., "Biological Action of Leptin as an Angiogenic Factor," *Science* 281, no. 5383 (September 11, 1998): 1683–86.

R. Strumia, E. Varotti, E. Manzato, and M. Gualandi, "Skin Signs in Anorexia Nervosa," *Dermatology* 203, no. 4 (2001): 314–17.

R. Strumia, "Dermatologic Signs in Patients with Eating Disorders," *American Journal of Clinical Dermatology* 6, no. 3 (2005): 165–73.

P. Fernández-Riejos et al., "Role of Leptin in the Activation of Immune Cells," *Mediators of Inflammation* 2010 (2010), Article ID: 568343, 8 pages.

J. Cason et al., "Cell-Mediated Immunity in Anorexia Nervosa," *Clinical & Experimental Immunology* 64, no. 2 (May 1986): 370–75.

E. Polack et al., "Low Lymphocyte Interferon-Gamma Production and Variable Pro- liferative Response in Anorexia Nervosa Patients," *Journal of Clinical Immunology* 13, no. 6 (November 1993): 445–51.

A. F. Osman et al., "The Incremental Prognostic Importance of Body Fat Adjusted Peak Oxygen Consumption in Chronic Heart Failure," *Journal of the American College of Cardiology* 36, no. 7 (December 2000): 2126–31.

M. R. Carnethon, et al., "Association of Weight Status with Mortality in Adults with Incident Diabetes," *Journal of the American Medical Association* 308, no. 6 (August 8, 2012): 581–90.

C. E. Hastie, "Obesity Paradox in a Cohort of 4880 Consecutive Patients Undergo- ing Percutaneous Coronary Intervention," *European Heart Journal* 31, no. 2 (2010): 222–26.

Stuart MacDonald, "Fat heart patients 'live longer,'" *The Sunday Times*, January 30, 2010.

4. When Good Fat Goes Bad

G. S. Hotamisligil, N. S. Shargill, and B. M. Spiegelman, "Adipose Expression of Tumor Necrosis Factor-Alpha: Direct Role in Obesity-Linked Insulin Resis- tance," *Science* 259, no. 5091 (January 1, 1993): 87–91.

S. P. Weisberg et al., "Obesity Is Associated with Macrophage Accumulation in Adi- pose Tissue," *Journal of Clinical Investigation* 112, no. 12 (December 15, 2003): 1796–1808.

H. Xu et al., "Chronic Inflammation in Fat Plays a Crucial Role in the Development of Obesity-Related Insulin Resistance," *Journal of Clinical Investigation* 112, no. 12 (December 15, 2003): 1821–30.

Y. Matsuzawa, S. Fujioka, K. Tokunaga, and S. Tarui. "Classification of Obesity with Respect to Morbidity," *Proceedings of the Society for Experimental Biology and Medicine* 200, no. 2 (June 1992): 197–201.

Y. Matsiizawa et al., "Visceral Fat Accumulation and Cardiovascular Disease," *Obe- sity Research* 3, S5 (December 1995): 645S–47S.

C. A. Slentz et al., "Inactivity, Exercise, and Visceral Fat. STRRIDE: a Randomized, Controlled Study of Exercise Intensity and Amount," *Journal of Applied Physiology* 99, no. 4 (October 2005): 1613–18.

B. A. Irving et al., "Effect of Exercise Training Intensity on Abdominal Visceral Fat and Body Composition," *Medicine and Science in Sports and Exercise* 40, no. 11 (November 2008): 1863–72.

P. E. Scherer et al., "A Novel Serum Protein Similar to C1q, Produced Exclusively in Adipocytes," *Journal of Biological Chemistry* 270, no. 45 (November 10, 1995): 26746–49.

A. H. Berg et al., "The Adipocyte-Secreted Protein Acrp30 Enhances Hepatic Insulin Action," *Nature Medicine* 7, no. 8 (August 2001): 947–53.

W. L. Holland et al., "The Pleiotropic Actions of Adiponectin Are Initiated via Receptor-Mediated Activation of Ceramidase Activity," *Nature Medicine* 17, no. 1 (January 2011): 55–63.

5. How Fat Fights to Stay on You

R. L. Leibel and J. Hirsch, "Diminished Energy Requirements in Reduced-Obese Patients," *Metabolism* 33, no. 2 (February 1984): 164–70.

M. Rosenbaum, J. Hirsch, D. A. Gallagher, and R. L. Leibel, "Long Term Persistence of Adaptive Thermogenesis in Subjects Who Have Maintained a Reduced Body Weight," *American Journal of Clinical Nutrition* 88, no. 4 (October 2008): 906–12.

M. Rosenbaum et al., "Low-Dose Leptin Reverses Skeletal Muscle, Autonomic and Neuroendocrine Adaptations to Maintenance of Reduced Weight," *Journal of Clinical Investigation* 115, no. 12 (December 2005): 3579–86.

M. Rosenbaum, J. Hirsch, E. Murphy, and R. L. Leibel, "Effects of Changes in Body Weight on Carbohydrate Metabolism, Catecholamine Excretion, and Thyroid Function," *American Journal of Clinical Nutrition* 71, no. 6 (June 2000): 1421–32.

M. Rosenbaum et al., "Low Dose Leptin Administration Reverses Effects of Sustained Weight Reduction on Energy Expenditure and Circulating Concentrations of Thyroid Hormones," *Journal of Endocrinology and Metabolism* 87, no. 5 (May 2002): 2391–94.

D. M. Thomas et al., "Why Do Individuals Not Lose More Weight from an Exercise Intervention at a Defined Dose? An Energy Balance Analysis," *Obesity Reviews* 13, no. 10 (October 2012): 835–47.

M. Rosenbaum et al., "Energy intake in weight reduced humans," *Brain Research* 1350 (September 2, 2010): 95–102.

M. Rosenbaum et al., "Leptin Reverses Weight Loss-Induced Changes in Regional Neural Activity Responses to Visual Food Stimuli," *Journal of Clinical Investigation* 118, no. 7 (July 2008): 2583–91.

P. Sumithran, et al., "Long-Term Persistence of Hormonal Adaptations to Weight Loss," *New England Journal of Medicine* 365, no. 17 (October 27, 2011): 1597–604.

The American Physiological Society Press Release, April 23, 2013, http://www.the-aps.org/mm/hp/Audiences/Public-Press/2013/14.html.

T. L. Hernandez et al., "Fat Redistribution Following Suction Lipectomy: Defense of Body Fat and Patterns of Restoration," *Obesity* 19, no. 7 (July 2011): 1388–95.

F. Benatti et al., "Liposuction Induces a Compensatory Increase of Visceral Fat Which Is Effectively Counteracted by Physical Activity: A Randomized Trial," *Journal of Clinical Endocrinology and Metabolism* 97, no. 7 (July 2012): 2388–95.

S. Taheri et al., "Short Sleep Duration Is Associated with Reduced Leptin, Elevated Ghrelin, and Increased Body Mass Index," *PLoS Medicine* 1, no. 3 (December 2004): e62, http://journals.plos.org/plosmedicine/article?id=10.1371/journal.pmed.0010062.

A. Everard and P. D. Cani, "Gut Microbiota and GLP-1," *Reviews in Endocrine and Metabolic Disorders* 15, no. 3 (September 2014): 189–96.

R. L. Batterham et al., "Critical Role for Peptide YY in Protein-Mediated Satiation and Body-Weight Regulation," *Cell Metabolism* 4, no. 3 (September 2006): 223–33.

Rexford Ahima, ed., *Metabolic Basis of Obesity* (New York: Springer-Verlag, 2011), pp. 110–12.

6. Bacteria and Viruses—Microscopic in Size, Giant in Effect

N. V. Dhurandhar et al., "Transmissibility of Adenovirus-Induced Adiposity in a Chicken Model," *International Journal of Obesity* 25, no. 7 (July 2001): 990–96.

N. V. Dhurandhar et al., "Association of Adenovirus Infection with Human Obesity," *Obesity Research* 5, no. 5 (September 1997): 464–69.

R. L. Atkinson et al., "Human Adenovirus-36 Is Associated with Increased Body Weight and Paradoxical Reduction of Serum Lipids," *International Journal of Obesity* 29, no. 3 (March 2005): 281–86.

N. V. Dhurandhar et al., "Human Adenovirus Ad-36 Promotes Weight Gain in Male Rhesus and Marmoset Monkeys," *Journal of Nutrition* 132, no. 10 (October 2002): 3155–60.

M. Pasarica et al., "Adipogenic Human Adenovirus Ad-36 Induces Commitment, Differentiation, and Lipid Accumulation in Human Adipose-Derived Stem Cells," *Stem Cells* 26, no. 4 (April 2008): 969–78.

E. M. Laing et al., "Adenovirus 36, Adiposity, and Bone Strength in Late-Adolescent Females," *Journal of Bone and Mineral Research* 28, no. 3 (March 2013): 489–96.

W.-Y. Lin et al., "Long-Term Changes in Adiposity and Glycemic Control Are Associated with Past Adenovirus Infection," *Diabetes Care* 36, no. 3 (March 2013): 701–7.

J. D. Voss et al., "Adenovirus 36 Antibodies Associated with Clinical Diagnosis of Overweight/Obesity but Not BMI Gain: A Military Cohort Study," *Journal of Clinical Endocrinology and Metabolism* 99, no. 9 (September 2014): e1708–12.

F. Bäckhed et al., "The Gut Microbiota as an Environmental Factor That Regulates Fat Storage," *Proceedings of the National Academy of Sciences of the United States of America* 101, no. 44 (November 2, 2004): 15718–23.

V. Ridaura et al., "Cultured Gut Microbiota from Twins Discordant for Obesity Modulate Adiposity and Metabolic Phenotypes in Mice," *Science* 341, no. 6150 (September 6, 2013).

T. S. Stappenbeck, L. V. Hooper, and J. I. Gordon, "Developmental Regulation of Intestinal Angiogenesis by Indigenous Microbes via Paneth Cells," *Proceedings of the National Academy of Sciences of the United States of America* 99, no. 24 (November 26, 2002): 15451–55.

R. E. Ley, P. J. Turnbaugh, S. Klein, and J. I. Gordon, "Microbial Ecology: Human Gut Microbes Associated with Obesity," *Nature* 444 (December 21, 2006): 1022–23.

P. J. Turnbaugh et al., "An Obesity-Associated Gut Microbiome with Increased Capacity for Energy Harvest," *Nature* 444 (December 21, 2006): 1027–31.

P. J. Turnbaugh et al., "A core gut microbiome in obese and lean twins," *Nature* 457 (January 22, 2009): 480–84.

E. Le Chatelier et al., "Richness of human gut microbiome correlates with metabolic markers," *Nature* 500 (August 29, 2013): 541–46.

P. J. Turnbaugh, F. Bäckhed, L. Fulton, and J. I. Gordon, "Diet-Induced Obesity Is Linked to Marked but Reversible Alterations in the Mouse Distal Gut Microbiome," *Cell Host Microbe* 3, no. 4 (April 17, 2008): 213–23.

A. Everard and P. D. Cani, "Gut Microbiota and GLP-1," *Reviews in Endocrine and Metabolic Disorders* 15, no. 3 (September 2014): 189–96.

E. van Nood et al., "Duodenal Infusion of Donor Feces for Recurrent *Clostridium Difficile*," *New England Journal of Medicine* 368, no. 5 (January 31, 2013): 407–15.

7. I Blame My Parents—Genes in Obesity

E. Ravussin et al., "Effects of a Traditional Lifestyle on Obesity in Pima Indians," *Diabetes Care* 17, no. 9 (September 1994): 1067–74.

L. O. Schulz et al., "Effects of Traditional and Western Environments on Prevalence of Type 2 Diabetes in Pima Indians in Mexico and the U.S.," *Diabetes Care* 29, no. 8 (August 2006): 1866–71.

Robert Pool, *Fat: Fighting the Obesity Epidemic* (New York: Oxford University Press, 2001).

L. Pérusse et al., "Familial Aggregation of Abdominal Visceral Fat Level: Results from the Quebec Family Study," *Metabolism* 45, no. 3 (March 1996): 378–82.

C. Bouchard et al., "The Response to Exercise with Constant Energy Intake in Identical Twins," *Obesity Research* 2, no. 5 (September 1994): 400–410.

C. Bouchard et al., "Response to Long Term Overfeeding in Twins," *New England Journal of Medicine* 322, no. 21 (May 24, 1990): 1477–82.

C. Bouchard et al., "Genetic Effect in Resting and Exercise Metabolic Rates," *Metabolism* 38, no. 4 (April 1989): 364–70.

A. Tremblay, J. A. Simoneau, and C. Bouchard, "Impact of Exercise Intensity on Body Fatness and Skeletal Muscle Metabolism," *Metabolism* 43, no. 7 (July 1994): 814–18.

J. E. Cecil et al., "An Obesity-Associated FTO Gene Variant and Increased Energy Intake in Children," *New England Journal of Medicine* 359, no. 24 (December 11, 2008): 2558–66.

M. Claussnitzer et al., "FTO Obesity Variant Circuitry and Adipocyte Browning in Humans," *New England Journal of Medicine* 373, no. 10 (September 3, 2015): 895–907.

T. O. Kilpeläinen et al., "Genetic Variation near IRS1 Associates with Reduced Adiposity and an Impaired Metabolic Profile," *Nature Genetics* 43, no. 8 (June 26, 2011): 753–60.

T. O. Kilpeläinen et al., "Physical Activity Attenuates the Influence of FTO Variants on Obesity Risk: A Meta-Analysis of 218,166 Adults and 19,268 Children," *PLoS Medicine* 8, no. 11 (November 2011): E1001116, http://journals.plos.org/plos medicine/article?id=10.1371/journal.pmed.1001116.

8. I Am Woman, I Have Fat

G. Rodríguez et al., "Gender Differences in Newborn Subcutaneous Fat Distribution," *European Journal of Pediatrics* 163, no. 8 (August 2004): 457–61.

W. W. K. Koo, J. C. Walters, and E. M. Hockman, "Body Composition in Human Infants at Birth and Postnatally," *Journal of Nutrition* 130, no. 9 (September 2000): 2188–94.

C. P. Hawkes, et al., "Gender- and Gestational Age-Specific Body Fat Percentage at Birth," *Pediatrics* 128, no. 3 (September 2011): e645–51.

J. Rigo et al., "Reference Values of Body Composition Obtained by Dual Energy

X-Ray Absorptiometry in Preterm and Term Neonates," *Journal of Pediatric Gastroenterology and Nutrition* 27, no. 2 (August 1998): 184–90.

A. J. O'Sullivan, "Does Oestrogen Allow Women to Store Fat More Efficiently? A Biological Advantage for Fertility and Gestation," *Obesity Reviews* 10, no. 2 (March 2009): 168–77.

W. C. Chumlea et al., "Body Composition Estimates from NHANES III Bioelectrical Impedance Data," *International Journal of Obesity and Related Metabolic Disorders* 26, no. 12 (December 2002): 1596–1609.

L. Davidsen, B. Vistisen, and A. Astrup, "Impact of the Menstrual Cycle on Determinants of Energy Balance: A Putative Role in Weight Loss Attempts," *International Journal of Obesity* 31, no. 12 (December 2007): 1777–85.

A. J. O'Sullivan, A. Martin, and M. A. Brown, "Efficient Fat Storage in Premenopausal Women and in Early Pregnancy: A Role for Estrogen," *Journal of Clinical Endocrinology and Metabolism* 86, no. 10 (October 2001): 4951–56.

B. N. Wu and A. J. O'Sullivan, "Sex Differences in Energy Metabolism Need to Be Considered with Lifestyle Modifications in Humans," *Journal of Nutrition and Metabolism* 2011 (2011), article ID: 391809.

G. N. Wade and J. M. Gray, "Gonadal Effects on Food Intake and Adiposity: A Metabolic Hypothesis," *Physiology and Behavior* 22, no. 3 (March 1979): 583–93.

L. E. Kopp-Hoolihan, M. D. van Loan, W. W. Wong, and J. C. King, "Longitudinal Assessment of Energy Balance in Well-Nourished, Pregnant Women," *American Journal of Clinical Nutrition* 69, no. 4 (April 1999): 697–704.

O. Koren et al., "Host Remodeling of the Gut Microbiome and Metabolic Changes During Pregnancy," *Cell* 150, no. 3 (August 3, 2012): 470–80.

P. Deurenberg, M. Deurenberg-Yap, and S. Guricci, "Asians Are Different from Caucasians and from Each Other in Their Body Mass Index/Body Fat Per Cent Relationship," *Obesity Reviews* 3, no. 3 (August 2002): 141–46.

P. T. Katzmarzyk et al., "Racial Differences in Abdominal Depot-Specific Adiposity in White and African American Adults," *American Journal of Clinical Nutrition* 91, no. 1 (January 2010): 7–15.

S. Nielsen et al., "Energy Expenditure, Sex, and Endogenous Fuel Availability in Humans," *Journal of Clinical Investigation* 111, no. 7 (April 2003): 981–88.

L. A. Anderson, P. G. McTernan, A. H. Barnett, and S. Kumar, "The Effects of Androgens and Estrogens on Preadipocyte Proliferation in Human Adipose Tissue: Influence of Gender and Site," *Journal of Clinical Endocrinology and Metabolism* 86, no. 10 (October 2001): 5045–51.

M. L. Power and J. Schulkin, "Sex Differences in Fat Storage, Fat Metabolism, and the Health Risks from Obesity: Possible Evolutionary Origins," *British Journal of Nutrition* 99, no. 5 (May 2008): 931–40.

E. J. Giltay and L. J. G. Gooren, "Effects of Sex Steroid Deprivation/Administration on Hair Growth and Skin Sebum Production in Transsexual, Males and Females," *Journal of Clinical Endocrinology and Metabolism* 85, no. 8 (August 2000): 2913–21.

J. M. H. Elbers et al., "Effects of Sex Steroids on Components of the Insulin Resistance Syndrome in Transsexual Subjects," *Clinical Endocrinology* 58, no. 5 (May 2003): 562–71.

M. J. Toth, A. Tchernof, C. K. Sites, and E. T. Poehlman, "Menopause-Related Changes in Body Fat Distribution," *Annals of the New York Academy of Sciences* 904 (May 2000): 502–6.

S. M. Byrne, Z. Cooper, and C. G. Fairburn, "Psychological Predictors of Weight Regain in Obesity," *Behaviour Research and Therapy* 42, no. 11 (November 2004): 1341–56.

9. Fat Can Listen

J. P. McNamara, "Role and Regulation of Metabolism in Adipose Tissue During Lactation," *Journal of Nutritional Biochemistry* 6, no. 3 (March 1995): 120–29.

M. Rebuffé-Scrive et al., "Fat Cell Metabolism in Different Regions in Women: Effect of Mentrual Cycle, Pregnancy, and Lactation," *Journal of Clinical Investigation* 75, no. 6 (June 1985): 1973–76.

Gareth Williams and Gema Fruhbeck, eds., *Obesity: Science to Practice* (Hoboken, NJ: Wiley-Blackwell, 2009).

P. Cuatrecasas, "Interaction of Insulin with the Cell Membrane: The Primary Action of Insulin," *Proceedings of the National Academy of Sciences of the United States of America* 63, no. 2 (June 1969): 450–57.

———, "Insulin-Receptor Interactions in Adipose Tissue Cells: Direct Measurement and Properties," *Proceedings of the National Academy of Sciences of the United States of America* 68, no. 6, (June 1971): 1264–68.

S. Bhasin et al., "The Effects of Supraphysiologic Doses of Testosterone on Muscle Size and Strength in Normal Men," *New England Journal of Medicine* 335, no. 1 (July 4, 1996): 1–7.

T. W. Burns et al., "Pharmacological Characterizations of Adrenergic Receptors in Human Adipocytes," *Journal of Clinical Investigation* 67, no. 2 (February 1981): 467–75.

I. Smilios et al., "Hormonal Responses After Resistance Exercise Performed with Maximum and Submaximum Movement Velocities," *Applied Physiology, Nutrition, and Metabolism* 39, no. 3 (March 2014): 351–57.

B. C. Nindl et al., "Twenty-Hour Growth Hormone Secretory Profiles After Aerobic and Resistance Exercise," *Medicine and Science in Sports and Exercise* 46, no. 10 (October 2014): 1917–27.

A. D. Kriketos et al., "Exercise Increases Adiponectin Levels and Insulin Sensitivity in Humans," *Diabetes Care* 27, no. 2 (February 2004): 629–30.

T. J. Saunders et al., "Acute Exercise Increases Adiponectin Levels in Abdominally Obese Men," *Journal of Nutrition and Metabolism* 2012 (2012), article ID: 148729.

L. A. Leiter, M. Grose, J. F. Yale, E. B. Marliss, "Catecholamine Responses to Hypocaloric Diets and Fasting in Obese Human Subjects," *American Journal of Physiology* 247, no. 2, pt. 1 (August 1, 1984): E190–97.

K. Y. Ho et al., "Fasting Enhances Growth Hormone Secretion and Amplifies the Complex Rhythms of Growth Hormone Secretion in Man," *Journal of Clinical Investigation* 81, no. 4 (April 1988): 968–75.

S. Taheri et al., "Short Sleep Duration Is Associated with Reduced Leptin, Elevated Ghrelin, and Increased Body Mass Index," *PLoS Medicine* 1, no. 3 (December 2004): e62, http://journals.plos.org/plosmedicine/article?id=10.1371/journal.pmed.0010062.

K. Spiegel, E. Tasali, P. Penev, and E. Van Cauter, "Sleep Curtailment in Healthy Young Men Is Associated with Decreased Leptin Levels, Elevated Ghrelin Levels, and Increased Hunger and Appetite," *Annals of Internal Medicine* 141, no. 11 (December 2004): 846–50.

R. L. Batterham et al., "Critical Role for Peptide YY in Protein-Mediated Satiation and Body-Weight Regulation," *Cell Metabolism* 4, no. 3 (September 2006): 223–33.

K. L. Knutson, "Does Inadequate Sleep Play a Role in Vulnerability to Obesity?," *American Journal of Human Biology* 24, no. 3 (May 2012): 361–71.

P. T. Williams, "Evidence for the Incompatibility of Age-Neutral Overweight and Age-Neutral Physical Activity Standards from Runners," *American Journal of Clinical Nutrition* 65, no. 5 (May 1997): 1391–96.

M. J. Cartwright, T. Tchkonia, and J. L. Kirkland, "Aging in Adipocytes: Potential Impact of Inherent, Depot-Specific Mechanisms," *Experimental Gerontology* 42, no. 6 (June 2007): 463–71.

10. Fat Control I: How You Can Do It

D. Zeevi et al., "Personalized Nutrition by Prediction of Glycemic Responses," *Cell* 163, no. 5 (November 19, 2015): 1079–94.

A. D. Kriketos et al., "Exercise Increases Adiponectin Levels and Insulin Sensitivity in Humans," *Diabetes Care* 27, no. 2 (February 2004): 629–30.

L. J. Goodyear and B. B. Kahn, "Exercise, Glucose Transport, and Insulin Sensitivity," *Annual Review of Medicine* 49 (February 1998): 235–61.

E. R. Ropelle et al., "IL-6 and IL-10 Anti-Inflammatory Activity Links Exercise to Hypothalamic Insulin and Leptin Sensitivity Through IKKb and ER Stress Inhibition," *PLoS Biology* 8, no. 8 (August 24, 2010): e1000465.

D. J. Dyck, "Leptin Sensitivity in Skeletal Muscle Is Modulated by Diet and Exercise," *Exercise and Sport Sciences Reviews* 33, no. 4 (October 2005): 189–94.

K. Y. Ho et al., "Fasting Enhances Growth Hormone Secretion and Amplifies the Complex Rhythms of Growth Hormone Secretion in Man," *Journal of Clinical Investigation* 81, no. 4 (April 1988): 968–75.

G. Frühbeck et al., "Regulation of Adipocyte Lipolysis," *Nutrition Research Reviews* 27, no. 1 (June 2014): 63–93.

M. L. Hartman et al., "Augmented Growth Hormone (GH) Secretory Burst Frequency and Amplitude Mediate Enhanced GH Secretion During a Two-Day Fast in Normal Men," *Journal of Clinical Endocrinology and Metabolism* 74, no. 4 (April 1992): 757–65.

A. F. Muller et al., "Ghrelin Drives GH Secretion During Fasting in Man," *European Journal of Endocrinology* 146, no. 2 (February 2002): 203–7.

J. E. Ahlskog, Y. E. Geda, N. R. Graff-Radford, and R. C. Petersen, "Physical Exercise as a Preventive or Disease-Modifying Treatment of Dementia and Brain Aging," *Mayo Clinic Proceedings* 86, no. 9 (September 2011): 876–84.

L. Davidsen, B. Vistisen, and A. Astrup, "Impact of the Menstrual Cycle on Determinants of Energy Balance: A Putative Role in Weight Loss Attempts," *International Journal of Obesity* 31, no. 12 (December 2007): 1777–85.

R. R. Wing and J. O. Hill, "Successful Weight Loss Maintenance," *Annual Review of Nutrition* 21 (2001): 323–41.

R. R. Wing and S. Phelan, "Long-Term Weight Loss Maintenance," *American Journal of Clinical Nutrition* 82, no. S1 (July 2005): 222S–225S.

M. L. Butryn, V. Webb, and T. A. Wadden, "Behavioral Treatment of Obesity," *Psychiatric Clinics of North America* 34, no. 4 (December 2011): 841–59.

J. G. Thomas et al., "Weight Loss Maintenance for 10 Years in the National Weight Control Registry," *American Journal of Preventive Medicine* 46, no. 1 (January 2014): 17–23.

11. Mind over Fat

Ancel Keys, Josef Brozek, Austin Henschel, Olaf Mickelsen, and Henry Longstreet Taylor, *The Biology of Human Starvation* (Minneapolis: University of Minnesota Press, 1950).

L. M. Kalm and R. D. Semba, "They Starved So That Others Be Better Fed: Remembering Ancel Keys and the Minnesota Experiment," *Journal of Nutrition* 135, no. 6 (June 1, 2005): 1347–52.

M. Rosenbaum et al., "Leptin Reverses Weight Loss-Induced Changes in Regional Neural Activity Responses to Visual Food Stimuli," *Journal of Clinical Investigation* 118, no. 7 (July 2008): 2583–91.

M. Muraven, "Building Self-Control Strength: Practicing Self-Control Leads to Improved Self-Control Performance," *Journal of Experimental Social Psychology* 46, no. 2 (March 1, 2010): 465–68.

L. H. Sweet et al., "Brain Response to Food Stimulation in Obese, Normal Weight, and Successful Weight Loss Maintainers," *Obesity* 20, no. 11 (November 2012): 2220–25.

S. M. McClure, D. I. Laibson, G. Lowenstein, and J. D. Cohen, "Separate Neural Systems Value Immediate and Delayed Monetary Rewards," *Science* 306, no. 5695 (October 15, 2004): 503–7.

T. Bradford Bitterly, Robert Mislavsky, Hengchen Dai, and Katherine L. Milkman, "Want–Should Conflict: A Synthesis of Past Research," in *The Psychology of Desire*, ed. Wilhelm Hoffman and Loran Nordgren (New York: Guilford Press, 2015).

H. Dai, K. L. Milkman, D. A. Hofmann, and B. R. Staats, "The Impact of Time at Work and Time Off from Work on Rule Compliance: The Case of Hand Hygiene in Health Care," *Journal of Applied Psychology* 100, no. 3 (May 2015): 846–62.

M. Muraven and R. F. Baumeister, "Self-Regulation and Depletion of Limited Resources: Does Self-Control Resemble a Muscle?," *Psychological Bulletin*, 126, no. 2 (March 2000), 247–59.

R. F. Baumeister, E. Bratslavsky, M. Muraven, and D. M. Tice, "Ego Depletion: Is the Active Self a Limited Resource?," *Journal of Personality and Social Psychology* 74, no. 5 (May 1998): 1252–65.

D. M. Tice, R. F. Baumeister, D. Shmueli, and M. Muraven, "Restoring the Self: Positive Affect Helps Improve Self-Regulation Following Ego Depletion," *Journal of Experimental Social Psychology* 43 (2007): 379–84.

Christine Haughney, "When Economy Sours, Tootsie Rolls Soothe Souls," *New York Times*, March 23, 2009.

K. L. Milkman, "Unsure What the Future Will Bring? You May Overindulge: Uncertainty Increases the Appeal of Wants over Shoulds," *Organizational Behavior and Human Decision Processes* 119, no. 2 (November 2012) 163–76.

M. Muraven, D. M. Tice, and R. F. Baumeister, "Self-Control as Limited Resource: Regulatory Depletion Patterns," *Journal of Personality and Social Psychology* 74, no. 3 (March 1998): 774–89.

G. Charness and U. Gneezy, "Incentives to Exercise," *Econometrica* 77, no. 3 (May 2009), 909–31.

12. Fat Control II: How I Do It

K. Van Proeyen et al., "Training in the Fasted State Improves Glucose Tolerance During Fat-Rich Diet," *Journal of Physiology* 588, pt. 21 (November 1, 2010): 4289–302.

M. A. Alzoghaibi, S. R. Pandi-Perumal, M. M. Sharif, and A. S. BaHammam, "Diurnal Intermittent Fasting During Ramadan: The Effects on Leptin and Ghrelin Levels," *PLoS One* 9, no. 3 (March 17, 2014): e92214.

13. The Future of Fat

P. A. Zuk et al., "Multi-Lineage Cells from Human Adipose Tissue: Implications for Cell-Based Therapies," *Tissue Engineering* 7, no. 2 (April 2001): 211–26.

S. Lendeckel et al., "Autologous Stem Cells (Adipose) and Fibrin Glue Used to Treat Widespread Traumatic Calvarial Defects: Case Report," *Journal of Cranio-Maxillo-Facial Surgery* 32, no. 6 (December 2004): 370–73.

C. Di Bella, P. Farlie, and A. J. Penington, "Bone Regeneration in a Rabbit Critical-Sized Skull Defect Using Autologous Adipose-Derived Cells," *Tissue Engineering. Part A* 14, no. 4 (April 2008): 483–90.

E. Alt et al., "Effect of Freshly Isolated Autologous Tissue Resident Stromal Cells on Cardiac Function and Perfusion Following Acute Myocardial Infarction," *International Journal of Cardiology* 144, no. 1 (September 24, 2010): 26–35.

S. S. Collawn et al., "Adipose-Derived Stromal Cells Accelerate Wound Healing in an Organotypic Raft Culture Model," *Annals of Plastic Surgery* 68, no. 5 (May 2012): 501–4.

C. Nie et al., "Locally Administered Adipose-Derived Stem Cells Accelerate Wound Healing Through Differentiation and Vasculogenesis," *Cell Transplant* 20, no. 2 (2011): 205–16.

Fred Tasker, "Patients Own Fat Cells Plump up Face, Breasts, Buttocks," *Miami Herald*, September 2, 2011.

Brett Flashnick, "Doctors Wary of Perry's Stem Cell Treatment," Associated Press, August 20, 2011, http://www.boston.com/news/nation/articles/2011/08/20/doctors _wary_of_perrys_stem_cell_treatment/?page=full.

INDEX

abstinence violation effect, 187
Ad-36 virus, 108–9, 110–11, 113
adipocytes. *see* fat cells
adiponectin
  exercise and, 72, 156, 167
  and insulin response, 71–72, 129,
    156
  and IRS1 gene, 129
  production and secretion by fat, 45,
    71–72, 73, 149, 156
  role in fat distribution, 45, 72, 129,
    167
adiponutrin, 45
adipose. *see* fat tissue (adipose tissue)
adipose derived stem cells (ASCs),
  202–4
adipsin, 45
adrenaline, 81, 84, 85, 86, 149, 157, 168
adrenaline receptors, 149
advertising, 2, 5
age and aging
  antiaging medicine, 155
  estrogen decrease, 140, 148, 149–50,
    193
  exercise effects and age, 159–60
  growth hormone decrease, 154, 155,
    193
  hormone replacement therapy, 154–
    56
  and physiology of fat, 147–48, 159–
    61

  testosterone decrease, 148, 149–50,
    152, 154, 155, 193
  thyroid hormone decrease, 154
Ajinkya, S. M., 100
Akkermansia muciniphila, 120
Allen, Frederick, 205
Alley, Kirstie, 6
Alstrom's syndrome, 27
Alt, Eckhard, 203
androgens, 52, 53, 56, 140
  see also testosterone
angiogenesis, 57–59, 90
angioplasty, 61
anorexia nervosa, 54, 55, 57, 59, 60
antiaging medicine, 155
Arnold, Donna, 203
aromatase, 52, 56
Aronne, Louis, 177
Atkinson, Richard, 105–6, 108, 109–
  11, 113, 177
Atwater, Wilbur, 4

Bäckhed, Fredrik, 115
bacteria and obesity
  Akkermansia muciniphila, 120
  bacterial transfer/transplant, 116,
    120, 135
  Bacteroidetes, 118, 120
  diversity and fat, 117–18
  FIAF (Fasting-Induced Adipose Fac-
    tor), 117

bacteria and obesity (*continued*)
  Firmicutes, 117–18, 119
  gut bacteria and obesity, 114–19,
    135, 197
  twin studies, 116–17
  see also viruses and obesity
Bacteroidetes, 118, 120
ballet dancers and menstruation,
  49–50, 51
Bardet-Biedl syndrome, 27
bariatric surgery, 63, 73, 74–75,
  113–14
Baumeister, Roy, 182
behavior therapy, 144, 206
beige fat, 21, 127
Benatti, Fabiana, 91
Berkman, Lisa, 48
The Biggest Loser (TV show), 6, 196
birth-control pills, 152, 158
Bishop, Katharine Scott, 24
blood sugar, normal level, 12
BMI (body mass index)
  and brain volume, 57
  and dementia risk, 57
  and fertility, 54–55
  genes linked to, 128
  mortality and, 60–62, 160
  normal levels, 54
  social conventions, 145
  and type 2 diabetes, 72
bone mineral density (BMD), 55
bone strength and development,
  55–56
Boorde, Andrew, 15
Botticelli, 3
Bouchard, Claude, 124–26, 128,
  167
BPA, 158, 159
Brady, Diamond Jim, 3
brain, 18, 56–57
brown fat
  activation of, 204–5
  in babies, 147
  cold temperatures and shivering,
    204–5
  distribution in body, 20

excessive amounts of, 22–23
  exercise effects, 21, 127, 168, 205
  from fat-derived stem cells, 204
  FGF21 emission, 204–5
  heat production, 20, 147, 168
  insulin sensitivity increased by, 23,
    204
  mitochondria in, 20
  transplantation in mice, 204
Buddha, 3
bulimia, 54
Burr, George, 23–25
Burr, Mildred, 24–25

calories, defined and introduced, 4
calories, efficient storage in fat, 18
Cani, Patrice, 119
canine distemper virus (CDV), 104,
  105, 106, 113
cardiopulmonary stress testing, 60
Carnethon, Mercedes, 61
cells, discovery of, 15
CELO virus, 108
ceramides, 72
changing views of fat, 1–7, 205–7
Charness, Gary, 188
Chehab, Farid, 52
chocolate cravings, 173–74
cholecystokinin (CCK), 88, 89, 93
cholesterol
  in cell membranes, 23
  decrease with Ad-36 virus, 108
  decrease with SMAM-1 virus, 101,
    102, 108
  normal level in blood, 12
chromosomes, 35–37, 40, 124
Claussnitzer, Melina, 127
Clostridium difficile, 120
Cohen, Jonathan, 184
Coleman, Douglas
  education, 29
  hypothesis about *ob* gene, 30, 31–32,
    34, 38, 40–41, 71
  Lasker Award, 42
  ob/db mouse research, 29–30, 31–32,
    34, 40

collagen, 15
cortisol, 27, 69, 149, 159
Cross, Marcia, 200
Cuatrecasas, Pedro, 148
Cushing's syndrome, 27, 80
cytokines, 68, 69

Dance Your A** Off (TV show), 6
Dansinger, Michael, 75, 168–69, 175–76, 195
Darnell, James, 33
db mice, 29–30, 31–32, 40–41, 42, 58
Dhurandhar, Nikhil
  Ad-36 virus, 108–9, 110–11, 112–13
  obtaining postdoctoral positions in America, 103–6
  SMAM-1 virus, 100–102
  weight loss program, 102, 110–11, 177
  youth and early career, 98–100
Dhurandhar, Vinod, 98
diabetes
  adiponectin deficiency, 72
  complications, 65
  effect of weight loss, 75–76
  obesity and, 64–65, 66, 67, 69
  treatment, 73, 76, 205–6
  type 2 diabetes, 63, 64, 69, 72, 129–30
Diabetes Prevention Program (DPP), 174
Diabetic Exchange diet, 107
dichotomous thinking, 143–44, 174, 198
Diet and Health: With Key to the Calories (Peters), 4–5
DietTribe (TV show), 6
Dikhtyar, Kira, 200
dinitrophenol (DNP), 5
DNA (deoxyribonucleic acid) structure, 35
DNP (dinitrophenol), 5
Donnelly, Joseph, 138, 172
Drinking Man's Diet, 5
dyslipidemia, 129

Eckel, Robert, 91
eicosanoids, 25
endocrine system, fat as organ in, 2, 14, 42, 45
energy and fat, 11, 18
energy as currency, 17–18
energy from digested food, 17–19
estrogen
  age-related decrease, 140, 148, 149–50, 193
  and bone strength, 55–56
  changes during menstrual cycle, 135
  estrogen dominance after menopause, 150
  and fat distribution, 139–40
  in men, 137, 140, 152
  obesity effects on, 53–54
  production in fat, 52, 54, 55, 56, 140, 147, 150
  risks, 155
  transdermal estrogen, 152
  xenoestrogens, 158–59
estrogen blockers, 153
ethnicity and fat, 137
Evans, Herbert McLean, 23–24
exercise and its effects
  adiponectin and, 72, 156, 167
  age differences, 159–60
  ballet dancers and menstruation, 50
  beige fat conversion to brown fat, 21, 127, 168
  delayed menarche, 50–51
  effect on hormone levels, 156–57, 167–68
  gender differences, 137–39, 172–73
  genetics and, 125–26, 131, 167
  ghrelin, 138
  High Intensity Interval Training (HIIT), 169, 171, 197, 198–99
  hunger after exercise, 137–38, 156–57, 168–69, 172–73
  insulin sensitivity increased by, 168
  irisin production, 21, 204–5
  after liposuction, 91–92

exercise and its effects (*continued*)
    sumo wrestlers, 70–71, 72–73, 167
    vigorous or strenuous exercise
        effects, 126, 167
    visceral fat reduction, 62, 72, 167
Extreme Makeover: Weight Loss Edition
    (TV show), 6

Farooqi, Sadaf, 43–44, 59
fasting
    FIAF (Fasting-Induced Adipose Fac-
        tor), 117
    gender differences, 137, 171
    and hormone levels, 157, 170–71,
        195
    intermittent fasting, 157, 170–72,
        194–95, 196, 198
Fasting-Induced Adipose Factor
    (FIAF), 117
fat
    as an organ, 2, 11, 14, 40, 42, 45,
        165
    changing views of, 1–7, 205–7
    defined, 11
    see also specific topics
Fat Actress (TV show), 6
fat cells (adipocytes)
    creation by stem cells, 7, 55, 202,
        204
    discovery of, 15
    expansion of, 15
    hormone receptors, 148–49
    insulin effect on, 68–69, 148–49, 199
    leptin release by, 40
    ob gene expression in, 39, 40
    TNFα production, 67
fat control tactics
    author's methods, 194–201
    building self-control "muscles,"
        181–84
    food logs, 75, 176–77, 196, 201
    fresh starts, 185–86
    habits of successful dieters, 174–76
    individualized diet plans, 166–67
    intermittent fasting, 157, 170–72,
        194–95, 196, 198

long-term weight loss, maintaining,
    92–93
motivation and triggers for dieting,
    144, 175, 185–86
precommitment devices, 185
setting meaningful goals, 189–90
"should" self and "want" self, 183–84
temptation bundling, 184–85
weight-loss coaches and support
    groups, 175–76, 177–78
see also exercise and its effects;
    reduced-obese
Fat Man's Club, 3, 4
Fatoff, 5
fat synthesis, 7, 16, 18, 55
fat tissue (adipose tissue)
    angiogenesis in, 90
    communication with other tissues,
        26–45, 148
    components, 15–16
    crowding in, 68–69
    dietary fat storage, 18
    leptin release, 41, 148–49
    macrophages in fat tissues, 67–68
    ob gene expression in, 40
    triglycerides deposited, 16
fatty acids, 15, 16, 17, 18
fatty acid synthase, 110
fecal transplant, 120
Ferrante, Anthony, 67, 68
fertility
    body fat and fertility, 51–52, 54–55,
        147–48
    body fat and menarche, 49
    leptin and, 52–53
    male fertility and weight loss, 53
    male libido and caloric intake, 53
    obesity effects on, 53–54
    weight and puberty relationship,
        47–49, 53, 147
    see also gender and fat
FGF21, 204–5
FIAF (Fasting-Induced Adipose Fac-
    tor), 117
fiber in diet, 93, 119, 157, 170, 172,
    173, 196–97

Firmicutes, 117–18, 119

Flegal, Katherine, 61–62

fMRI (functional magnetic resonance imaging), 86, 181, 182, 184, 192–93

Folkman, Judah, 58–59, 90

food logs, 75, 176–77, 196, 201

Friedman, Jeffrey
  discovery of leptin, 41–42, 52
  education, 32–34
  Lasker Award, 42
  ob gene discovery and cloning, 40, 43
  search for *ob gene*, 33, 34, 36–37, 38–40, 71

Frisch, Henry, 51

Frisch, Rose
  ballet dancer research, 50
  body fat and fertility, 49–51, 54–55
  death, 54
  education, 46
  exercise and fertility, 50–51
  John Simon Guggenheim Memorial Foundation fellowship, 47
  weight and puberty relationship, 47–49

fructose, 170

FTO gene, 126–27, 128, 130–31, 193

functional magnetic resonance imaging (fMRI), 86, 181, 182, 184, 192–93

Galen, 15

García-Cardeña, Guillermo, 58

Gardner Reducing Machine, 5

gastric bypass surgery, 63, 113–14

gel electrophoresis, 28, 43

gender and fat, 132–45
  body building by women, 141–42
  changes in menopause, 140, 149–50
  fasting effects, 137
  fat distribution, 139–41
  Martha and Tom, 132–33, 145
  in newborns, 134
  nutrient partitioning, 136, 139, 173

pregnancy and weight gain, 135–36, 148

psychological differences, 142–45, 173–74

puberty, 47–49, 53, 134, 147

response to exercise, 137–39

why women get fatter than men, 133–37
see also fertility; menstruation

genes, overview, 35–36

genes in obesity
  effects of diet, 131
  exercise and genetics, 125–26, 131, 167
  FTO gene, 126–27, 128, 130–31, 193
  healthy obesity genes, 127–30
  IRS1 gene, 128–30
  overview, 121, 130–31, 165
  Pima Indians, 121–24, 130, 192
  thrifty genotype, 122, 123, 192
  twin studies, 125

Germans, overweight, 2

Ghadir, Shahin, 54

ghrelin, 88, 89, 92–93, 138, 157–58, 170–71

Gingrich, Newt, 1, 7

Glass, D. C., 188

GLP-1, 88, 89

glucose
  for current energy needs, 17
  high levels after meals, 18
  insulin effect on uptake, 68–69, 148–49
  insulin response to, 166, 170
  molecular structure, 17

glycemic index, 88

glycogen, 17, 18

Gneezy, Uri, 188

Gobley, Theodore, 15, 202

gonadotropin-releasing hormone, 52–53

Gordon, Jeffrey, 115–17, 118

Grapefruit Diet, 5

Gray, Martha, 132–33, 145

Greece, ancient beliefs about fat, 14–15

Green, Ariana, 146, 147, 150–52, 154,
    159
growth hormone, 149, 154, 155, 156–
    57, 170–71, 195
Gu, Jian-Wei, 90

Hamdy, Osama, 75–76
Hanson, Mike, 146–47, 152–53, 154,
    155, 159
Harris, Patrice, 206
Heaton, Patricia, 200
Heavy (TV show), 6
Helicobacter pylori, 112
Henry VIII (king), 15
Hernandez, Teri, 91
High Intensity Interval Training
    (HIIT), 169, 171, 197, 198–99
high pressure liquid chromatography,
    28
Hill, James, 174
Hippocrates, 15
Hirsch, Joy, 85–86, 180–81
Hirsch, Jules, 81–82
Hoffman, David, 54
hormone replacement therapy (HRT)
    antiaging medicine, 154–56
    growth hormone injections, 155
    leptin replacement therapy, 57, 60
    for menopausal women, 151, 155, 156
    risks, 155–56
    testosterone replacement therapy,
        155
    and weight loss, 151–52, 155–56
Hotamisligil, Gökhan, 65–67, 68
How To Be Plump, 3
human chorionic gonadotropin, 151
hunger, effects of prolonged, 179–81
Hussain, Khalid, 21–22

immune system
    activation by tumor necrosis factor
        alpha, 66–67
    anorexia nervosa effects, 60
    fat communication with, 65–69
    immune cells in fat, 67–68, 69
    leptin and, 59–60

infectobesity, 100, 112–13
inflammation, defined, 68
insulin
    adiponectin and, 71–72, 129, 156
    effect on fat cells, 68–69, 148–49,
        199
    hunger suppression, 197
    obesity effects on, 53–54
    release from pancreas, 18, 68
    response to carbohydrate intake,
        166, 170
    sensitivity increased by brown fat,
        23, 204
    sensitivity increased by exercise, 168
    sugar and fat uptake by cells, 68–69,
        148–49
    TNFα interference with signaling,
        66
insulin receptors, 148–49
insulin resistance, 66–67, 68–69
intermittent fasting, 157, 170–72,
    194–95, 196, 198
irisin, 21, 204–5
IRS1 gene, 128–30
I Used to Be Fat (TV show), 6

Jenny Craig, 6
Jensen, Michael, 134, 136, 137–39,
    144–45, 173, 193
Jerry, 158–59
Joyce, Sarah, 51

Keys, Ancel, 179–80, 195
Kilpeläinen, Tuomas, 128
Kreek, Mary Jeanne, 33

Ladies Home Journal, 3
La Mar Reducing Soap, 5
Lancha, Antonio, 91
Lavie, Carl, 60–61, 62
Lee, Paul, 204–5
Leibel, Rudolph (Rudy)
    and childhood obesity, 79–80,
        86–87
    early career, 79–81, 85–86, 87
    macrophages in fat tissues, 67

metabolism of reduced-obese,
81–86, 87–88, 89, 90, 92, 144
search for *ob* gene, 36, 81
Lendeckel, Stefan, 203
leptin
and adrenaline, 85
angiogenesis promotion, 58–59
appetite suppression, 40, 42, 43, 52,
86, 170
binding to hypothalamus, 42
decreased levels in reduced-obese,
84–85, 181
defect in *ob* mice, 41, 42
discovery, 41–42, 52
fasting effects on, 195
and fat metabolism, 44
and fertility, 52–53
fructose and leptin resistance, 170
gonadotropin-releasing hormone
activation, 52–53
and immune system, 59–60
injections for reduced-obese, 87, 181
lipodystrophy and, 19, 42
measurement in blood, 43
and noradrenaline, 85
obesity effects on, 53–54
from *ob* gene, 40–41
and psychological maturity, 53
release by fat, 40–41, 148–49
and sexual maturation, 52–53, 147
and skeletal muscle energy use, 85, 86
sleep and, 92–93, 170, 195
and thyroid hormone, 85
and wound healing, 59
leptin receptors, 42, 58, 60
linoleic acid, 24–25
lipids, defined, 15
lipodystrophy, 12–14, 19–20, 42
lipogenesis, 18
lipolysis, 18
liposuction, 31, 90–92, 167, 202, 203
liver, functions of, 16, 17, 18
long-term weight loss, maintaining,
92–93
Look AHEAD (Action for Health in
Diabetes), 174

Loos, Ruth, 127–29, 130–31
Love Handles (TV show), 6
Lucky Strike Cigarettes, 5

MacDonald, Paul, 52
macrophages, 67–68
malfunctioning fat, health effects, 19
Malik, Layla, 26–27, 31, 37–38,
43–45, 87, 130
Marshall, Barry, 112
Matsuzawa, Yuji, 70–71
Maugh, Kathy, 63–65, 69, 73–75,
76–77
McClure, Samuel, 184
McConaughey, Matthew, 200
McQuillan, Sharon, 203
menstruation
anorexia nervosa and, 54
ballet dancers, 49–50, 51
body fat and, 49–51, 147
bulimia and, 54
changes in appetite and fat storage,
135, 173–74
see also gender and fat
metformin, 73, 76
microbiome
correlation within family, 115, 192
defined, 117
and diet, 119–20, 172, 196–97
diversity and fat, 117–18, 172
gut bacteria and obesity, 114–19,
135, 197
microdissection, 36–37, 38
Milkman, Katherine, 183–84, 186,
187
miscarriage and body weight, 54
mitochondria in brown fat, 20
Mohammed, Shehla, 37–38
money spent fighting fat, 2
money spent on weight loss product
ads, 2
motivation and triggers for dieting,
144, 175, 185–86
Muraven, Mark, 181–82, 183, 184,
187, 189
myelin, 23

National Health and Nutrition Exam-
ination Survey (NHANES),
134–35
National Institute of Diabetes and
Digestive and Kidney Diseases
(NIDDK), 122–23, 196
National Weight Control Registry
(NWCR), 168, 174, 175, 182,
190, 201
neuropathy, 65, 69
Nindl, Bradley, 156
Nishi, Kai, 73–74, 75, 76–77
noradrenaline, 84, 85, 86
nutrient partitioning, 136, 139, 173
Nutrisystem, 6

obesity
    crowding in fat tissue, 68–69
    and diabetes, 64–65, 66, 67, 69
    effects on estrogen, 53–54
    and infertility, 53–54
    number of obese Americans, 2
    recognition as a disease, 206
    see also genes in obesity; reduced-
        obese
obesity paradox, 60–62, 160
ob gene
    discovery and cloning, 40, 43
    expression in fat cells, 39, 40
    molecular control of behavior, 33, 45
    mutations in humans, 43–44
    search for gene, 33, 34–35, 36–37,
        38–40, 71
ob mice (*ob/ob* mice)
    defective leptin in, 41, 42
    introduction, 28, 29
    model system of obesity, 28
    molecular control of behavior, 33, 34
    parabiosis with *db* mice, 30
    reduced brain weight and volume,
        56
oligofructose, 119, 172
One Big Happy Family (TV show), 6
O'Rahilly, Stephen, 37–38, 43–45, 59
Oral, Elif, 13
osteocalcin, 56

O'Sullivan, Anthony, 136–37, 138,
    139, 152
Overton, Charles Ernest, 23

Palmer, Colin, 126, 127
Papapetropoulos, Andreas, 58
paraben, 158
parabiosis, 30
Pell, Jill, 61
peptide YY (PYY), 88, 89, 93
Perry, Rick, 203
Peters, Lulu Hunt, 4
phthalates, 158, 159
physiological functions of fat
    age differences, 147–48, 159–61
    body fat and fertility, 51–52, 54–55,
        147–48
    bone development, 55–56
    brain size, 56–57
    in cell membranes, 23
    disease survival, 60–62
    fat as messenger, 23–25
    immune system, 57–62, 65
    male fertility and weight loss, 53
    menarche and body fat, 49
    menstruation and body fat, 49–51,
        147
    milk and lactation, 136, 148
    obesity effects on fertility, 53–54
    overview, 2–3, 7
    reserve energy storage, 11, 18
    signaling molecules, 23–25, 65
    weight and puberty relationship,
        47–49, 53, 147
    see also specific types of fat
Pima Indians, 121–24, 130, 192
plasmapheresis, 14, 19–20
Power, Karron, 154–55, 156, 158–59,
    169
Prader-Willi syndrome, 27
prebiotics, 119–20
precommitment devices, 185
pregnancy and weight gain, 135–36,
    148
probiotics, 119
proconvertase-1 hormone, 37–38

progesterone, 135, 148, 149–50
Proietto, Joseph, 87–89, 192
prostaglandins, 25
Proteus syndrome, 65–66

Randall, 78–80, 81, 86–87
Randy
  antibodies to Ad-36, 110
  boyhood, 97–98
  diabetes, 106–7
  efforts to control weight, 98, 102–3,
    107, 109–10, 113–14, 177–78, 191
  scratched by chicken, 97, 98, 111
Ravussin, Eric, 123–24
reduced-obese
  altered hormone levels, 84–85, 89,
    181
  decreased calorie requirements, 82,
    83, 84, 86, 92
  description, 82
  fMRI brain images, 85–86, 180–81,
    182, 192–93
  increased drive to eat, 85–86, 89,
    165, 181
  leptin injections, 87, 181
  leptin levels decreased in, 84–85,
    181
  research design, 83, 88–89
  see also obesity
resistin, 45
retinol binding protein-4, 45
Revelle, Roger, 47, 48
Rhees, Jocelyn, 21–23
Ridaura, Vanessa, 116
Rittenberg, David, 16, 202
Rosenbaum, Michael
  about, 82
  brain activity in dieters, 85–86,
    180–81
  metabolism of reduced-obese,
    82–85, 87–88, 89, 92, 144, 192
Roth, J. D., 6
Rous-associated virus (RAV), 104, 113
rubber suits for weight loss, 5
Rubens, 3
Russell, Lillian, 3, 4

Sandra, 78–80
Scherer, Phil, 71–72
Schneider, Bruce, 33
Schoenheimer, Rudolph, 16, 202
Segal, Eran, 166, 196
self-control
  abstinence violation effect, 187
  building self-control "muscles,"
    181–84
  fatigue from overusing self-control,
    186–87
  fMRI scans of brain activity, 182,
    184
  fresh starts, 185–86
  precommitment devices, 185
  setting meaningful goals, 189–90
  "should" self and "want" self, 183–
    84
  temptation bundling, 184–85
  uncertainty and stress effects, 188–
    89
  see also fat control tactics
sex hormone binding globulin
  (SHBG), 152, 158, 159
Shapiro, Benyamin, 16
Shedding for the Wedding (TV show),
  6
Sherrod, Drury, 188
Sierra-Honigmann, Rocío, 58–59
Siiteri, Pentti, 52
Sisson, Mark, 171
sleep and hormone levels, 92–93,
  157–58, 170, 195
SMAM-1 virus, 100–102, 103, 107–8,
  192
Spiegelman, Bruce, 21
Sputnik, 28
Stanford, Kristin, 204
starvation, effects of, 179–81
stem cells
  adipose derived stem cells (ASCs),
    202–4
  creation of bone cells, 55
  creation of fat cells, 7, 55, 202, 204
  in fat tissue, 16, 202–3
stickK.com, 185

stretch receptors, 170
Stunkard, Albert, 99
subcutaneous fat
adiponectin effects, 72
benefits during sickness, 62
estrogen production, 52
IRS1 gene and, 129
liposuction effects, 91–92
puberty effects, 134
sumo wrestlers, 70–71, 72–73, 167

Taft, Howard, 4
Tang Dynasty in China, 3
tapeworms, 5
temptation bundling, 184–85
The 10 Most Fascinating People of 1995
(television show), 1
Terry, 176
testosterone
age-related decrease, 148, 149–50,
152, 154, 155, 193
exercise effect on, 156
and fat distribution, 139, 148, 152
lean muscle mass promotion, 152,
154
leptin and, 53
risks, 155
testosterone cycle, 152, 154
in women, 148, 150, 152
see also androgens
testosterone stimulators, 153
thermogenin, 20
thrifty genotype of Pima Indians, 122,
123, 192
thyroid hormone, 27, 84, 85, 86, 154
Tice, Dianne, 187
Titian, 3
Tobias, Jonathan, 56
Tokmakidis, Savvas, 156
Treat and Reduce Obesity Act, 206
Tremblay, Angelo, 126
triglycerides
decrease with Ad-36 virus, 108
decrease with SMAM-1 virus, 101,
102, 108
deposition in fat tissue, 16, 90

fatty acids in, 18
molecular structure, 16, 17, 18
normal level in blood, 12
tumor necrosis factor alpha (TNFα),
66–67, 68
type 2 diabetes, 63, 64, 69, 72,
129–30

U.S. Department of Homeland Security, 2

van Leeuwenhoek, Antonie, 15, 25,
114
Vena, Christina, 11–14, 19–20, 42
Vincent, Lawrence, 49–50
viruses and obesity
Ad-36 virus, 108–9, 110–11, 113
canine distemper virus (CDV), 104,
105, 106, 113
Rous-associated virus (RAV), 104,
113
skepticism about viruses and fat,
111–13
SMAM-1 virus, 100–102, 103,
107–8, 192
vaccines and, 113
see also bacteria and obesity
visceral fat
and brain health, 57, 69
defined, 57, 69
exercise and, 62, 72, 167
genetics and, 125
health risks, 69, 140
inflammation and, 62, 140
IRS1 gene and, 129
after liposuction, 91–92
menopause and, 140
oligofructose and, 119
sumo wrestlers and, 70–71, 73, 167
visfatin, 45
vitamin E, 24
Vodianova, Natalia, 200

Wadden, Thomas, 176
Walters, Barbara, 1, 7
Warren, Robin, 112

weight control tactics. *see* fat control
    tactics
Weight Watchers, 6
Weisberg, Stuart, 67
Wertheimer, Haim Ernst, 16
white fat, 20, 21, 127, 147, 165, 204–5
Williams, Paul, 160
will power. *see* self-control
Winfrey, Oprah, 7

Wing, Rena, 174–75, 182
Winslow, Sherry, 141–43, 144, 189
wound healing and leptin, 59
Wyshak, Grace, 48

xenoestrogens, 158–59
X-ray absorptiometry, 115

Zuk, Patricia, 202–3